Medicine

NOTICE

Medicine is an ever-changing science. As new research and clinical experience broaden our knowledge, changes in treatment and drug therapy are required. The editors and the publisher of this work have made every effort to ensure that the drug dosage schedules herein are accurate and in accord with the standards accepted at the time of publication. Readers are advised, however, to check the product information sheet included in the package of each drug they plan to administer to be certain that changes have not been made in the recommended dose or in the contraindications for administration. This recommendation is of particular importance in regard to new or infrequently used drugs.

Medicine:
PreTest® Self-Assessment and Review

Second Edition

Edited by
John M. Dwyer, M.D., Ph.D.
Associate Professor of Medicine
Yale University School of Medicine
New Haven, Connecticut

Associate Editor
Denis J. Miller, M.D.
Associate Professor of Medicine
Yale University School of Medicine
New Haven, Connecticut

McGraw-Hill Book Company
Health Professions Division
PreTest Series

New York St. Louis San Francisco Auckland Bogotá Guatemala Hamburg Johannesburg Lisbon London Madrid Mexico Montreal New Delhi Panama Paris São Paulo Singapore Sydney Tokyo Toronto

Library of Congress Cataloging in Publication Data
Main entry under title:

Medicine: PreTest self-assessment and review.
First ed. (1978) edited by John M. Dwyer.
Bibliography: p.
1. Medicine – Examinations, questions, etc.
I. Dwyer, John M. II. Miller, Denis J. [DNLM:
1. Medicine – Examination questions. W18 M5113]
R834. 5.M4 1981 616'.0076 80-23823

ISBN 0-07-050971-9

6 7 8 9 0 HUHU 8 7 6 5 4

Editor: *John H. Gilchrist*
Project Editor: *Aaron E. Klein*
Editorial Assistant: *Donna Altieri*
Production: *Rosemary J. Pascale, Judith M. Raccio*
Designer: *Robert Tutsky*
Printer: *Hull Printing Company*
Cover Illustration: *Sir William Osler at the Bedside. From a photograph, courtesy of Oxford University Press.*

Contents

List of Contributors

Joseph R. Bloomer, M.D.
Professor of Medicine
Dight Institute
University of Minnesota School of Medicine
Minneapolis, Minnesota

Robert L. Capizzi, M.D., F.A.C.P.
Professor of Medicine and Pharmacology
Chief, Division of Medical Oncology
University of North Carolina School of Medicine
Chapel Hill, North Carolina

Richard J. Dean, M.D.
Attending Urologist
Yale-New Haven Hospital
New Haven, Connecticut

John M. Dwyer, M.D., Ph.D.
Associate Professor of Medicine
Yale University School of Medicine
New Haven, Connecticut

John A. Hardin, M.D.
Associate Professor of Medicine
Yale University School of Medicine
New Haven, Connecticut

Robert L. Marier, M.D.
Associate Professor of Medicine
Louisiana State University
New Orleans, Louisiana

William W. Merrill, M.D.
Assistant Professor of Medicine
Yale University School of Medicine
New Haven, Connecticut

Denis J. Miller, M.D.
Associate Professor of Medicine
Yale University School of Medicine
New Haven, Connecticut

James J. Nordlund, M.D.
Associate Professor of Dermatology
Yale University School of Medicine
New Haven, Connecticut

Lawrence A. Reduto, M.D.
Fellow in Cardiology
Yale-New Haven Hospital
New Haven, Connecticut

David Satinsky, M.D.
Associate Clinical Professor of Neurology
George Washington University
School of Medicine and Health Sciences
Washington, D.C.

Robert Sherwin, M.D.
Associate Professor of Medicine
Yale University School of Medicine
New Haven, Connecticut

Introduction

Medicine: PreTest® Self-Assessment and Review has been designed to provide students, as well as physicians, with a comprehensive and convenient instrument for self-assessment and review within the field of medicine. The 500 questions provided have the same format and are of the same degree of difficulty as the questions contained in Part II of the National Board of Medical Examiners examinations, the Federation Licensing Examination (FLEX), the Visa Qualifying Examination, and the ECFMG examination.

Each question in the book is accompanied by an answer, a paragraph explanation, and a specific page reference to either a current journal article, a textbook, or both. A seven page bibliography, listing all the sources used in the book, follows the last chapter.

Perhaps the most effective way to use this book is to allow yourself one minute to answer each question in a given chapter; as you proceed, indicate your answer beside each question. By following this suggestion, you will be approximating the time limits imposed by the board examinations previously mentioned.

When you finish answering the questions in a chapter, you should then spend as much time as you need verifying your answers and carefully reading the explanations. Although you should pay special attention to the explanations for the questions you answered incorrectly, you should read **every** explanation. The authors of this book have designed the explanations to reinforce and supplement the information tested by the questions. If, after reading the explanations for a given chapter, you feel you need still more information about the material covered, you should consult and study the references indicated.

This book is intended to be educative as well as evaluative; we hope that you enjoy it. We also would be happy to receive your comments.

Preface

The usefulness of realistically testing one's knowledge prior to examination is obvious. Periodic self-assessment, however, should surely be as normal a part of continuing education for medical practitioners as general reading and attendance at conferences. The second edition of *Medicine: PreTest Self-Assessment and Review* should be of considerable help to medical students, residents, and physicians in this respect. In the new questions supplied for this edition, we have concentrated more on clinical problems at both the diagnostic and therapeutic level and somewhat less on pathogenic mechanisms. We have reviewed leading articles published in some of the major medical journals over the past three years and have made certain that questions highlighting newer information are included. Information pertinent to the answer to every question in the book can be found in the standard textbooks of medicine and we have given specific pagination to the ninth edition of *Harrison's Principles of Internal Medicine.* In many situations, however, we felt that more detailed information would be needed and references to either journal articles or sections of subspecialty textbooks are included.

We have presented all of the questions to medical students prior to the completion of their studies to ascertain that no questions are too difficult or too easy. The standard of the questions, however, has been deliberately graded in conformity with the examination questions mentioned in the Introduction to the book. The questions in the second edition have been specifically chosen so that, in following up the answers given, the reader will be led into important and related areas of medicine that were not possible to explore in this book. For example: following up a question on one of the types of hyperlipidemia naturally would lead to variations in this disorder that one might expect to encounter.

Having used this book extensively in teaching exercises with medical students, the Editors find that the questions – in the format presented – offer a sort of lighthearted challenge that can be the ideal way for introducing a discussion of a given topic. Thus, we are hopeful that this book will have a wide appeal to students and clinicians anxious to keep their knowledge of internal medicine up-to-date.

J.M.D.
D.J.M.

Allergy and Immunology

DIRECTIONS: Each question below contains five suggested answers. Choose the **one best** response to each question.

1. Plasmapheresis is used in the management of such diseases as myasthenia gravis, systemic lupus erythematosus, and idiopathic thrombocytopenic purpura. Which of the following statements about this form of therapy is true?

(A) It is used only when hypergammaglobulinemia is present
(B) It is hazardous in patients with anemia
(C) It is of little use in patients receiving prednisone or immunosuppressive agents
(D) It is effective only in adults
(E) It can produce clinical improvement in less than 24 hours

2. Which of the following statements about thymus-derived lymphocytes (T lymphocytes) is true?

(A) Malignant proliferation of T lymphocytes is the major feature of acute lymphatic leukemia in children
(B) T lymphocytes provide the first line of defense against viral infection
(C) The function of T lymphocytes is readily suppressed by steroids
(D) T lymphocytes have a lifespan in excess of four years
(E) Twenty percent of the lymphocytes in peripheral blood are T lymphocytes

3. Immunologic reactions to tumor-specific antigens have been demonstrated in a number of human malignancies. In such cases, which of the following statements is true?

(A) The lymphocytes of nonaffected individuals are more cytotoxic for the tumor cells than those of affected patients
(B) The sera of affected patients frequently can kill the patients' own lymphocytes in culture
(C) Affected patients' immune complexes (tumor-specific antigens and antibodies to tumor-specific antigens) may block T-cell antitumor responses
(D) Affected patients' T cells must release lymphokines to activate complement pathways for a successful tumoricidal response
(E) Immunotherapy with BCG vaccine is thought to enhance tumor destruction by increasing circulating levels of cytotoxic antibody

4. Alpha-methyldopa (Aldomet) may cause an autoimmune hemolytic anemia. This complication is associated with

(A) the development of high titers of antinuclear factor
(B) a strongly positive indirect Coombs' (antiglobulin) test
(C) the development of an autoantibody with specificity for the Rh locus
(D) a slow but consistent reversal of the hemolytic process if the drug is withdrawn
(E) the binding of the drug to the red blood cell membrane, which produces an immunogenic hapten protein conjugate

5. Acquired hypogammaglobulinemia results in a marked increase in the frequency and severity of bacterial infections. Current evidence suggests that the pathogenesis of this disease may be related to

(A) the administration of gammaglobulin in the first few months of life
(B) failure of stem cell differentiation to B lymphocytes in the bone marrow
(C) a failure of helper T cells to collaborate with B lymphocytes in the production of antibody
(D) abnormally rapid shedding of B-cell receptors for antigen with subsequent poor recognition of an antigenic presence
(E) the abnormal activation of suppressor T cells that block B-cell production of an antibody secreting system

6. Selective IgA deficiency is the most common of all immunodeficiency states. Study of patients who have this problem has revealed that

(A) they may suffer anaphylactic reactions following the administration of serum products
(B) encouraging improvements in health follows regular infusions of fresh plasma
(C) secretory component is usually increased in an attempt to compensate for lack of secretory IgA
(D) there is an increase in 19S IgM in the secretions of certain affected patients
(E) a few of them may have associated autoimmune disorders

7. A 60-year-old man experiences a sudden onset of severe lower back pain; he gives a history of recent weight loss and a first attack of gout. An immunoelectrophoretic strip reveals a monoclonal gammopathy. Which of the following statements about this patient is most likely to be true?

(A) The monoclonal immunoglobulin will be of the IgM class
(B) Ten to 15 percent of the patient's bone marrow cells will be plasma cells
(C) A polyclonal increase in the immunoglobulin classes not involved in the gammopathy also will be present
(D) The patient's urine will contain large amounts of free monoclonal kappa chains
(E) Gammaglobulin therapy is unlikely to be of any help

8. Which of the following statements about allergic reactions in patients receiving up to 20 g of penicillin per day is true?

(A) Allergic reactions occur in 20 percent of patients receiving the drug for the second time
(B) Allergic reactions may be anaphylactoid if IgE class antibodies to penicilloyl-P are present in the serum
(C) Allergic reactions will be less likely to occur if IgM antipenicilloyl antibodies are present in the serum
(D) Allergic reactions are unlikely to be anaphylactoid if the patient does not get a wheal and flare reaction when penicilloyl-D-lysine is introduced intradermally
(E) Allergic reactions can be complicated by hemolytic anemias when prolonged administration provokes the development of red blood cell autoantibodies

9. Which of the following statements about assessment of immunoglobulin in cerebrospinal fluid is true?

(A) It may aid in the diagnosis of cerebral systemic lupus erythematosus
(B) It may lead to a suspicion of multiple sclerosis if IgM levels are elevated
(C) It may distinguish subacute sclerosing panencephalitis from multiple sclerosis
(D) It normally reveals that five to ten percent of the cerebrospinal fluid protein is IgG
(E) It becomes more useful if the total cerebrospinal fluid protein exceeds 100 mg/100 ml

10. A 24-year-old woman who is investigated by an endocrinology unit is discovered to have primary ovarian failure and diabetes. This syndrome would be expected to be associated with all the following factors EXCEPT

(A) premature graying of the hair
(B) vitiligo
(C) a mother with proven pernicious anemia
(D) antibodies reactive with salivary glands
(E) antibodies reactive with thyroglobulin

11. Immune complexes can produce severe pathologic reactions in such structures as blood vessels, joints, and basement membranes. Which of the following statements concerning the major mechanism actually causing the tissue damage is true?

(A) It results from the release of cytotoxic lymphokines from T cells triggered by the complexes
(B) It results from a direct cytotoxic effect of activated complement components $C\bar{5}$, $C\bar{6}$, and $C\bar{7}$
(C) It results from the release by tissue mast cells of slow-reacting substance of anaphylaxis, increasing vascular permeability
(D) It results from the release of lysosomal enzymes from polymorphonuclear leukocytes
(E) It can be blocked if sufficient vasoactive amines can be released from lysed platelets

12. Which of the following statements about the presence of circulating anti-deoxyribonucleoprotein in the serum of patients who have systemic lupus erythematosus is true?

(A) It is associated with the presence of LE cells
(B) It is associated with leukopenia since the antibody reacts with neutrophil membrane antigens
(C) It is rarely associated with high titers of antinuclear factor
(D) It is an indication that severe membranous glomerulonephritis is likely to be present
(E) It is unusual inasmuch as this antibody generally is associated with scleroderma

13. A one-year-old male child has a history of recurrent infections from low-grade pathogens since birth. He has chronic suppurative and granulomatous lesions of the skin and lymph nodes; his humoral and cellular immune system is intact. The child would be expected to have

(A) recurrent pneumococcal pneumonia that fails to resolve despite appropriate antibiotic therapy
(B) a father whose leukocytes demonstrate an impaired ability to reduce the dye nitroblue tetrazolium
(C) leukocytes with an increased ability to phagocytose catalase-positive bacteria
(D) a failure of normal hydrogen peroxide production in leukocytes that have ingested bacteria
(E) a marked reduction in the ability of phagocytes to produce lactate

14. A 15-year-old girl presents with a clinical syndrome that is indistinguishable from viral hepatitis; however, her history and serological findings do not support a viral etiology for her problem. Liver biopsy reveals an established active cirrhosis and hepatocellular necrosis associated with a heavy infiltrate of plasma cells and lymphocytes. Which of the following statements about this girl's condition is most likely to be true?

(A) B lymphocytes are likely to carry the histocompatibility antigen B7
(B) She probably has a total immunoglobulin level that exceeds 4 g/100 ml
(C) She probably has antimitochondrial antibodies
(D) High titers of antismooth muscle antibodies are likely to appear transiently at the onset of her illness
(E) She will probably recover spontaneously after six months of illness

15. The 6th chromosome in humans carries A, B, C, and D loci that contain genes whose products are detected as histocompatibility antigens on the surface of most cells in the body. The association of certain diseases with specific alleles at these loci may correctly be said to

(A) have been made possible by the development of mixed leukocyte reactions with pooled normal cells
(B) be best exemplified by the association of the B27 antigen with ankylosing spondylitis and psoriatic arthritis
(C) be explained by linkage dysequilibrium of these alleles to immunoregulatory alleles
(D) suggest that viruses can trigger certain diseases by utilizing these histocompatibility antigens as receptors through which to gain entry to cells
(E) occur much more frequently in women than in men

16. A 40-year-old man presents with a three-month history of headache, sinusitis, and rhinorrhea. He has had two episodes of hemoptysis and some respiratory discomfort. On examination, he has some nasal mucosal ulcerations. His blood urea nitrogen is 60 mg per 100 ml. A biopsy of the swollen tissue in the patient's nose yields results consistent with a diagnosis of Wegener's granulomatosis. All the following histological features can be expected to be associated with this condition EXCEPT for

(A) vasculitis affecting the small arterioles
(B) vasculitis involving venules and some capillaries
(C) deposition in blood vessels of immunoglobulin and, possibly, immune complexes
(D) necrotizing inflammation in which all affected vessels show the same degree of inflammation
(E) numerous giant cells in granulomata

DIRECTIONS: Each question below contains four suggested answers of which **one** or **more** is correct. Choose the answer:

A	if	**1, 2, and 3**	are correct
B	if	**1 and 3**	are correct
C	if	**2 and 4**	are correct
D	if	**4**	is correct
E	if	**1, 2, 3, and 4**	are correct

17. Mixed cryoglobulins have which of the following characteristics?

(1) They are frequently found in patients with systemic lupus erythematosus
(2) They are associated with low whole serum complement levels
(3) They are composed of relatively more IgG than IgM
(4) They are cryoprecipitable only in the presence of the 11S Clq component of complement

18. Hereditary angioneurotic edema is associated with which of the following statements?

(1) It results from the presence of abnormally high levels of IgE
(2) It is frequently associated with severe abdominal cramps
(3) It is sometimes associated with the release of massive amounts of histamine
(4) During an attack it is frequently associated with the consumption of the natural substrates for $C\bar{1}$, $C\bar{4}$, and $C\bar{2}$

19. Once activated, individual components of the classical pathway for complement are capable of

(1) enhancing polymorphonuclear cell phagocytosis
(2) lysing cell membranes
(3) interacting with kinin and fibrolytic systems
(4) neutralizing viruses

20. In comparing the immunologic features of tuberculoid leprosy to those of lepromatous leprosy, it is found that patients with lepromatous leprosy

(1) have much greater levels of circulating gamma globulin
(2) have a profound anergy to the antigenic determinants of *Mycobacterium leprae*
(3) frequently have a circulating factor that inhibits lymphocyte DNA synthesis
(4) are more prone to erythema nodosum reactions when treatment is instituted

21. A 24-year-old woman has a severe anaphylactic reaction following a honeybee sting. She recovers, but is surprised and disappointed at her reaction since she had completed a course of desensitization with whole-body extract. In discussing the future management of this problem, the physician would be correct in telling the patient that

(1) she should have a skin test with whole-body extract and, if the result is positive, she should try a second course of desensitizing injections with this antigenic preparation
(2) she should not be alarmed about the situation because, despite the fact that there are hundreds of thousands of bee stings a year in the United States, only 50-60 deaths are reported annually
(3) even if she is stung after another course of desensitization and no immediate reaction occurs, she should watch for a delayed reaction for at least two hours after the sting
(4) most reactions appear to occur because of sensitivity to bee and hornet venom

22. Correct statements about asthma (reversible airways obstruction) include which of the following?

(1) It is associated with deficient alpha-adrenergic receptor function
(2) It is frequently associated with respiratory syncytial virus infections early in life
(3) Affected patients suffering attacks in which P_{CO_2} levels remain normal are unlikely to require hospitalization
(4) It is associated with an increased bronchial sensitivity to slow-reacting substance of anaphylaxis and to bradykinin

23. Correct statements about hereditary ataxia-telangiectasia include which of the following?

(1) It is associated with the presence of congenital telangiectasias
(2) It is associated with a normal cell-mediated immunity but an absence or marked deficiency of IgA
(3) It is a syndrome transmitted in an X-linked mode
(4) Associated death commonly results from lymphoreticular malignancy in the second and third decade of life

SUMMARY OF DIRECTIONS

A	B	C	D	E
1, 2, 3 only	1, 3 only	2, 4 only	4 only	All are correct

24. Bone marrow-derived B lymphocytes exhibit which of the following characteristics?

(1) They are the proliferating cells in chronic lymphocytic leukemia
(2) They carry a surface membrane receptor for the Fc portion of IgG
(3) They carry a surface membrane receptor for breakdown products of the third component of complement
(4) They have a receptor for the Epstein-Barr virus

25. Antibodies that act as circulating anticoagulants demonstrate which of the following characteristics?

(1) They usually are IgM in character
(2) They increase rapidly in the serum after exposure to blood or blood products
(3) They may be present for years in apparently normal postpartum women
(4) In patients who have systemic lupus erythematosus, they are often directed against activated factor X

DIRECTIONS: The groups of questions below consist of lettered choices followed by several numbered items. For each numbered item select the **one** lettered choice with which it is **most** closely associated. Each lettered choice may be used once, more than once, or not at all.

Questions 26-29

For each of the following immunologic phenomena, select the immunologic agent with which it is most closely associated.

(A) $C\overline{8}$
(B) T cells
(C) IgG
(D) IgM
(E) IgE

26. Contact sensitivity
27. Allograft rejection
28. Arthus' reactions
29. Multiple myeloma

Questions 30-32

For each of the following immunologic techniques, select the immunologic factor with which it is most closely associated.

(A) T-cell cytotoxicity
(B) Quantitative IgA levels
(C) Monoclonal spikes
(D) B lymphocytes
(E) IgE

30. Gel diffusion
31. Radioimmunoassay
32. Chromium isotope release assays

Questions 33-35

Match the following.

(A) Secretory piece
(B) Germinal centers
(C) Cyclophosphamide
(D) IgA
(E) IgM

33. Intestinal epithelium
34. Bladder epithelium
35. Splenic vein

Questions 36-39

For each of the following disorders, select the feature with which it is most closely associated.

(A) C1 esterase inhibitor
(B) Peyer's patches
(C) Rheumatoid factor
(D) Allergic reactions to iodides
(E) Sympathetic ophthalmia

36. Rheumatoid arthritis
37. Systemic lupus erythematosus
38. Sjögren's syndrome
39. Leprosy

Allergy and Immunology Answers

1. The answer is E. *(Isbister, Med J Aust 2:167-170, 1979. Isselbacher, ed 9. p 359.)* Militant plasmapheresis is presently used in many clinical situations in which antibodies (e.g., antiplatelet or anticholinesterase receptor antibodies) or immune complexes (e.g., systemic lupus erythematosus, rheumatoid arthritis) are thought to be producing severe disease. It has been demonstrated that the removal of 4-8 liters of plasma per week can significantly lower circulating antibody/immune complex levels in adults. An affected patient frequently improves within hours after a single bleeding (e.g., improved muscle strength in myasthenia gravis, increased platelet count in idiopathic thrombocytopenic purpura). It is not necessary to achieve hypergammaglobulinemia and low complement levels prior to treatment. Improved technology allows considerable amounts of plasma to be removed, even from children. The problem of anemia that might occur with repeated bleedings is solved by replacement of red blood cells. B-cell clones producing antibodies involved in the pathogenesis of the disease being treated are stimulated to produce more antibodies after plasmapheresis, and at this time B cells are highly susceptible to cytotoxic drugs (e.g., cyclophosphamide).

2. The answer is D. *(Isselbacher, ed 9. pp 315-319.)* Thymus-derived lymphocytes are detected by the rosettes formed when the lymphocytes are exposed to red blood cells obtained from sheep. Once identified with this technique, the cells can be purified and studied. The human thymus produces lymphocytes from the 10th week of fetal life. The major period of thymus activity extends through fetal life into the first few years of postgestational life. Early atrophy of the thymus is compensated for by the extraordinary lifespan of T lymphocytes. In humans, individual lymphocytes may live for 60 years or more. The thymus gland produces at least four distinct types of T cells. These are: (1) immunoregulatory cells (suppressor cells) exercising control over all immunologic effector mechanisms (the immunologic thermostat); (2) helper T cells that allow bone marrow-derived B cells to produce IgG and IgA antibodies; (3) T cells that can produce delayed hypersensitivity; and (4) those that can kill antigenic target cells (cytotoxic T lymphocytes). In only 25 percent of cases of childhood acute lymphatic leukemia are the proliferating cells T cells. Effector T cells supply our major defense against fungi and intracellular bacteria, but antibodies supply the first line of defense against viruses by preventing the viral particles from entering cells. These cells, comprising 80 percent of the circulating lymphocytes, are resistant to steroids.

3. **The answer is C.** *(Eisen, pp 621-622. Isselbacher, ed 9. pp 1609, 1819-1820.)* Immunologic surveillance is a mechanism provided by T lymphocytes involving the recognition and destruction of proliferating clones of malignant cells. Malignant cells carry immunogenic tumor-specific antigens; the inability of T cells to recognize such antigens (e.g., in primary immune deficiency or in an immunosuppressed patient) is clearly associated with an increased risk of malignancy. Except in leukemias, beneficial cytotoxic antibodies are rare; it is usual to find blocking or enhancing antibodies or antigen-antibody complexes that hide tumor-specific antigen from the T cell. Immunotherapy with BCG is based on the demonstrated ability of such adjuvants to stimulate T-cell activity. Ideally, it should be coupled with procedures that reduce the level of blocking antibody. Lymphocytes from patients with tumors do frequently show an in vitro ability to destroy tumor cells, while cells from normal subjects do not. The serum from affected patients can frequently be shown to block destruction of malignant cells, but does not itself kill the patients' lymphocytes.

4. **The answer is C.** *(Gell, ed 3. pp 939-941. Isselbacher, ed 9. pp 1533-1545.)* Alpha-methyldopa leads to the development of a positive direct Coombs' test in 20 percent of patients receiving this hypotensive agent. The drug induces an autoantibody directed against the Rh locus and may cause frank hemolysis. Rapid reversal of the syndrome occurs with drug withdrawal or steroid therapy. The drug does not bind more strongly to red blood cells of affected patients than of normal individuals. Antinuclear factor is not found in patients receiving alpha-methyldopa, but is found with drug reactions to procainamide. A mechanism similar to that seen with alpha-methyldopa has been reported following therapy with levodopa and mefenamic acid.

5. **The answer is E.** *(Bach, pp 787-789. Isselbacher, ed 9. pp 320-330.)* Acquired hypogammaglobulinemia is a severe disease in which minimal antibody production is associated with an increased propensity for bacterial infection. Acquired hypogammaglobulinemia differs from congenital agammaglobulinemic states in that B lymphocytes are usually present in normal numbers, with normal receptors for antigen. There is no evidence for a failure of stem cell differentiation as a cause of acquired hypogammaglobulinemia. Recent studies strongly suggest that, in at least one-third of affected patients, B cells fail to respond to antigen because of active restraints imposed by patients' own immunoregulatory T cells

acting in an exaggerated manner. B lymphocytes, when freed from the presence of T cells, can produce normal amounts of antibody. Some patients increase their antibody production when treated with steroids. The mechanism is unknown, but, since suppressor T cells are sensitive to steroids, these drugs may be suppressing "suppressor" cells.

6. **The answer is A.** *(Gell, ed 3. pp 200-202. Isselbacher, ed 9. pp 330-331.)* IgA deficiency occurs in approximately 1 out of 700 births. Failure to produce this antibody results in recurrent upper respiratory tract infections in 50 percent of affected patients. IgA-deficient patients frequently have autoimmune disorders, atopic problems, and malabsorption, and eventually develop pulmonary disease. There is an increased incidence of malignancy in these cases. Replacement therapy is entirely unsatisfactory. If IgA is totally absent, its administration can represent an antigenic challenge that may result in anaphylaxis. Secretory component is normally present, and very few cases of IgA deficiency are due to a lack of this accessory factor. Some patients compensate for IgA deficiency by secreting a low molecular weight 7S IgM antibody.

7. **The answer is D.** *(Gell, ed 3. pp 397-398. Isselbacher, ed 9. pp 333-336.)* Multiple myeloma is a tumor in which there is malignant proliferation of a clone of plasma cells producing a homogeneous antibody product. Often there is a history of chronic infection, and some of the monoclonal antibodies have been found to react with bacterial antigens. The class of immunoglobulin involved is usually G or A and, as most human immunoglobulins carry kappa light chains, kappa chains are more frequently found in the urine as Bence Jones proteins than are lambda chains. Because the malignant cell does a poor job of linking together light and heavy chains, the light chains, having a low molecular weight, are filtered by the kidney. Humoral substances released by monocytes (probably with T-cell help) attempt to suppress the abnormal clone. They fail, but do suppress normal immunoglobulin production so that such patients frequently are functionally agammaglobulinemic and need replacement therapy with immunoglobulin.

8. **The answer is B.** *(Eisen, pp 583-585. Isselbacher, ed 9. p 384.)* Allergic reactions to penicillin consist of: (1) immediate hypersensitivity reactions; (2) delayed-immediate type hypersensitivity reactions; (3) delayed in-time reactions; and (4) delayed reactions involving organ specific tissue. The antigenic determinants of penicillin that provoke these reactions can be subdivided into minor and major determinants. The major determinants constitute the majority of the breakdown metabolites of penicillin and are represented by the penicilloyl

derivatives. It is the minor determinants, however, that produce most of the severe, immediate allergic reactions. Penicillin hypersensitivity is usually mediated by IgE and IgM antibodies against these metabolic degradation products of penicillin. With both the major and the minor determinants, it is necessary for the penicillin to form a conjugate with a body protein, inasmuch as the breakdown products of penicillin are not, in themselves, immunogenic. Such complexes are known as hapten protein conjugates. IgE antibody—usually against minor determinants—can produce the severe immediate anaphylactoid reactions that often are life threatening. Sensitivity to these minor determinants can only be predicted from a patient's history and from immediate hypersensitivity reactions to intradermal injection of the drug to be used. Minor determinant mixtures for skin testing are not commercially available. In some patients, however, IgE antibodies to the major (penicilloyl) determinants are present, and immediate hypersensitivity in the skin will occur following skin testing with penicilloyl. While most of the immediate (2-30 minutes) reactions are due to IgE antibody directed against minor determinants, reactions that begin within 3 hours and, perhaps, as late as 72 hours can be mediated by IgE against the penicilloyl derivatives. These are known as delayed-immediate hypersensitivity reactions. Delayed in-time reactions, which are intermediated by IgG antibodies, occur after 48 hours. The majority of penicillin reactions are caused by complement activation following IgM antibodies combining with major determinants. The hapten protein complexes are usually formed in the skin, which, therefore, become a frequent target for the reaction, although serum sickness-like disease may occur. Hemolytic anemia can occur if penicillin determinants form hapten protein conjugates with red blood cells. Antipenicillin antibodies react with the adsorbed penicillin, causing subsequent red blood cell lysis. No autoantibodies are formed in this condition. Allergic reactions may occur in as many as 10 percent of persons treated with penicillin, and there seems little doubt that IgG blocking antibodies prevent an even higher incidence of such reactions.

9. The answer is D. *(Isselbacher, ed 9. p 1975. Thompson, ed 2. p 101.)* Normally, IgG represents 5 to 10 percent of the total protein in cerebrospinal fluid. Levels exceeding 12 percent have been shown to correlate with the presence of either multiple sclerosis or subacute sclerosing panencephalitis. In other conditions, evaluations of cerebrospinal fluid immunoglobulin have not been valuable because the IgG fraction usually remains proportionate to the total level of cerebrospinal fluid protein. The discriminatory value of IgG determination is lessened once the level of total protein exceeds 100 mg/100 ml.

10. The answer is D. *(Fudenberg, ed 2. p 628. Isselbacher, ed 9. pp 321-323, 1711, 1782. MacKay, Postgrad Med 35:7-17, 1969.)* The patient presented in the question exhibits signs of the thyrogastric cluster of autoimmune diseases. These diseases feature autoantibodies directed against specific targets that are subsequently diseased or destroyed. This characteristic is in contrast to the lupus cluster of diseases in which immune complexes produce a vasculitis or the destruction of cell membranes through an immunologic reaction initiated by the immune complex. Diseases included in the thyrogastric cluster are: (1) primary ovarian failure, (2) hypoparathyroidism, (3) thyrotoxicosis, (4) Hashimoto's thyroiditis, (5) vitiligo, (6) diabetes, (7) primary adrenal failure, and (8) myasthenia gravis. Associated with the vitiligo is premature graying of the hair, defined for this purpose as half of the hairs on the head graying by the age of 30. Clustering is defined as the occurrence, in one patient, of more than one of these diseases or the occurrence of more than one of these diseases in the families of patients. Antibodies to the salivary glands can be found in Sjögren's syndrome but are not found in the thyrogastric cluster of diseases.

11. The answer is D. *(Eisen, pp 550-551. Isselbacher, ed 9. pp 347-351.)* Immune complexes trigger a chain reaction that involves the lysis of platelets and the release of vasoactive amines, the activation by steric changes in the Fc portion of IgG and IgM of the complement cascade, and the infiltration of polymorphonuclear leukocytes under the chemotactic influence of $C\bar{5}$, $C\bar{6}$, and $C\bar{7}$. Polymorphonuclear leukocytes release lysosomal enzymes that cause damage to cells alongside the complexes and local connective tissue elements.

12. The answer is A. *(Isselbacher, ed 9. pp 355-356. Stiehm, ed 2. p 521.)* Antideoxyribonucleoprotein (anti-DNP) antibody, one of the antinuclear factors found in the lupus erythematosus (LE) cluster of diseases, constitutes the LE factor that promotes phagocytosis of nuclear material by polymorphonuclear leukocytes to produce the LE cell. While the antibody is associated with lupus erythematosus, it is not as good a correlate of renal disease as is the presence of antideoxyribonucleic acid antibody. Antibodies to soluble nuclear extracts correlate better with scleroderma. Although individuals who have systemic lupus erythematosus can exhibit leukopenia and even an antibody to neutrophils, such phenomena are not particularly associated with anti-DNP antibody.

13. The answer is D. *(Isselbacher, ed 9. p 288. Park, pp 326-329.)* The child presented in the problem probably has chronic granulomatous disease. Frequently inherited by an X-linked pattern, the disease is associated with normal phagocytosis but an abnormal ability to produce hydrogen peroxide (H_2O_2), owing to a faulty hexose-monophosphate shunt. Because organisms that produce their own

H_2O_2 can still be killed by these leukocytes, problems with such organisms as pneumococcus and *Streptococcus* are not common. Leukocytes associated with chronic granulomatous disease cannot reduce the dye nitroblue tetrazolium, a diagnostic test. The disorder usually is fatal at an early age.

14. The answer is B. *(Gell, ed 3. pp 1277-1279. Isselbacher, ed 9. pp 1470-1472.)* The patient presented in the question probably has chronic active hepatitis, an autoimmune liver disease characterized by the chronic presence of anti-smooth muscle antibody and severe hypergammaglobulinemia. The disease usually is relentlessly progressive, developing eventual portal hypertension and episodes of bleeding. Antimitochondrial antibodies exist in 10 to 20 percent of affected patients but are more commonly associated with primary biliary cirrhosis. Chronic active hepatitis, which belongs to the lupus group of disorders, is infrequently associated with thyroid and gastric disorders. No consistent patterns relating HLA phenotypes and chronic active hepatitis have been found so far.

15. The answer is C. *(Isselbacher, ed 9. pp 360-365.)* A, B, and C-locus antigens are present on all cells in the body except red blood cells. D-locus antigens are most strongly expressed in B lymphocytes and macrophages. The antigens are detected by antisera specific for each allele. The cumbersome mixed lymphocyte reaction formerly used to detect D locus antigens is being replaced by this serological technique. In animal models, the locus that is equivalent to the D locus of humans has been found to be intimately associated with immune response and immunoregulatory genes. It seems likely that the association of a particular D-locus antigen with a disease reflects an affinity of these genes for specific genes that allow abnormal immune responses to occur (linkage dysequilibrium). The B27 antigen, which is found in 95 percent of patients with ankylosing spondylitis, is **not** associated with psoriatic arthritis; psoriasis is associated with the B13 and Bw17 antigens. B27 occurs with very high frequency in Reiter's syndrome and uveitis. Some antigens (e.g., B8), when associated with autoimmune disease, occur more frequently in women than men, although this is not true of HLA and disease associations in general.

16. The answer is D. *(Isselbacher, ed 9. pp 935-936.)* Necrotizing vasculitis is associated with a variety of conditions that cover the spectrum from leukocytoclastic angiitis (mild) to necrotizing midline granuloma (severe). Within this spectrum, a clinically definable constellation of clinical and pathological findings makes it possible to define the syndrome known as Wegener's granulomatosis. The therapeutic and prognostic implications of this syndrome make its diagnosis a matter of some importance. Wegener's granulomatosis is a systemic disease in which inflammation results from vasculitis occurring in many vessels throughout the body. Venules, capillaries, and arterioles are all affected in this disease, which is most commonly seen in men in the fourth and fifth decades of life. Characteristically, however, blood vessels in the kidneys and both upper and lower respiratory tracts are most affected. Although the evidence is not conclusive, there are data to suggest that the immune system produces this vasculitis as part of a hypersensitivity reaction to an antigenic encounter yet to be identified. Circulating immune complexes have been demonstrated in some, but not all, cases and granulomata are found in many tissues, observations that strengthen the concept of a hypersensitivity state and implicate cell-mediated immunity in the pathogenesis of the disease. Giant cell formation, probably representing fused macrophages, is often associated with the granulomata. The vasculitis associated with Wegener's granulomatosis is unusual in that careful examination of blood vessels in one tissue section will show some that are undergoing early inflammatory changes, others that are obviously healing, and still others that are permanently sclerosed.

17. The answer is E (all). *(Isselbacher, ed 9. p 336.)* Mixed cryoglobulins are frequently associated with systemic lupus erythematosus and diseases suspected to be of similar etiology. These cryoglobulins, which are most frequently found in patients who have comcomitant active disease, renal damage, and low total serum complement levels, invariably consist of IgG and IgM, with the former predominating. Alpha-2-macroglobulins are often included, and the macromolecular complex needs the 11S Clq complement component for cryoprecipitation to occur. The IgM moiety frequently has anti-IgG activity and is thus likened to a rheumatoid factor.

18. The answer is C (2, 4). *(Benacerraf, pp 238-239. Isselbacher, ed 9. pp 306, 356.)* Hereditary angioneurotic edema is a symptom complex involving attacks of laryngeal edema and interstitial swelling associated with rapid accumulation of edema fluid in nonpruritic lesions. The attacks may arise spontaneously but frequently occur following trauma, menses, exercise fatigue, and even psychologic stress. The disease is caused by genetically transmitted (autosomal dominant) defects in either the production or activity of the inhibitor for the first component of complement. Stimulation of the complement cascade is unchecked during the early steps of the reaction, and the excessive amount of activated complement components produces pharmacologic effects via a kinin-like substance, resulting in marked vasopermeability.

19. The answer is E (all). *(Isselbacher, ed 9. pp 322-323.)* At least eleven serum proteins interact in a chain reaction to provide the classical complement system. These chain reactions are activated by antigen-antibody complex formation in which the antibody is either of the IgM or three of the four subclasses of IgG. An alternate pathway that bypasses the first five steps of the classical pathway may be activated by, among other things, endotoxins and certain polysaccharides. The complement system amplifies inflammation in a nonspecific manner. Each component in the reaction, once activated, is biologically active. Among the major properties of the activated molecules are the ability to (1) dilate blood vessels and deliver cells to inflammatory sites, (2) chemotactically attract and activate polymorphonuclear cells, (3) lyse cell membranes, and (4) interact with the kinin, fibrinolytic, and coagulation systems. Excessive inflammation is avoided through deactivation of the components shortly after activation. The complement system is needed for most antibody mediated cytotoxic reactions. The consumption of components can exceed supply in severe immune complex diseases, such as systemic lupus erythematosus.

20. The answer is E (all). *(Isselbacher, ed 9. pp 711-714. Samter, ed 3. pp 627-638.)* Leprosy is a disease caused by *Mycobacterium leprae*. This acid-fast organism produces a spectrum of disease that ranges from a tuberculoid form to a lepromatous form. In the tuberculoid form, host defense mechanisms are able to contain the spread of the disease, apparently via a cell-mediated immune reaction. In lepromatous leprosy, the more serious form of the disease, a susceptible host's cell-mediated responses are overwhelmed, extensive destruction of lymphoid tissue occurs, and noncytotoxic antibodies are produced in abundance. With initiation of treatment (especially with sulfones), erythema nodosum occurs in 30 to 50 percent of both varieties of leprosy. It is not known what determines the form of the disease that these slow-growing organisms will take.

21. The answer is D (4). *(Hunt, J Allergy Clin Immunol 59:2-8, 1977. Isselbacher, ed 9. p 925.)* Desensitization of individuals who are hypersensitive to wasp and bee stings with whole-body hymenoptera extract has been successful in desensitizing some people but the efficacy of this treatment in most cases has been subject to question. Recent investigations have shown that the major antigenic determinant responsible for anaphylactic reactions is contained within the venom of stinging wasps, hornets, and bees. Desensitization with venoms obtained from the specific species to which a given patient is allergic produces reliable and measurable results. Although it is true that only a relatively small number of deaths due to hypersensitivity reactions is reported annually, these statistics have no bearing on an individual patient's situation. The danger for any given patient who has had an anaphylactoid reaction is very high. Many accidents occur annually when patients who know they are allergic to bee stings find themselves driving an automobile with a bee for a passenger. Patients should be taught how to use bee sting emergency kits containing epinephrine and should be counseled about the not-infrequent delayed reactions that occur after a sting. Reactions quite commonly occur after 24 hours and some reactions have been reported to start 48 hours after the stinging. Although desensitization with venom—as opposed to whole-body—extract is currently expensive, desensitization with these preparations is now the clear treatment of choice.

22. The answer is C (2, 4). *(Isselbacher, ed 9. pp 1201-1208. Stiehm, ed 2. pp 456-462, 681.)* Recent evidence suggests that asthma is associated with an imbalance in autonomic bronchial tone involving a deficiency in beta-adrenergic receptors. The relative increase in alpha-receptor influence establishes conditions for bronchospasm in response to a variety of stimuli. The bronchial tree of normal individuals receiving beta-adrenergic blockers becomes sensitive to histamine, slow-reacting substance of anaphylaxis, bradykinin, and acetylcholine. Asthmatic individuals not receiving such drugs are similarly sensitive. In children, respiratory syncytial virus frequently supplies a stimulus for bronchospasm. Because hyperventilation in asthma usually results in low P_{CO_2} levels, even normal levels suggest a very severe attack of asthma.

23. The answer is D (4). *(Isselbacher, ed 9. pp 329-330, 2008.)* Hereditary ataxia-telangiectasia is a syndrome transmitted in an autosomal recessive mode. It consists of cerebellar ataxia, pseudopalsy of eye movements developing during infancy, and conjunctival telangiectasias developing at five or six years of age. The immune defect consists of IgA deficiency (80 percent) and decreased cell-mediated immune functioning (100 percent). The thymus gland is poorly differentiated, and there is a depletion of the paracortical T-cell dependent areas of the lymph nodes.

24. The answer is E (all). *(Dwyer, Prog Allergy 21:182, 197, 212, 216, 1976. Isselbacher, ed 9. pp 315-316.)* B lymphocytes are cells that mature in the bone marrow and have surface receptors that bind the Fc portion of IgG, some complement components, the Epstein-Barr virus, and, most importantly, specific antigen. The latter is accomplished via a specific immunoglobulin receptor molecule. The cells have a short half-life (days) and are thus quite different from T cells that live for years. Oncogenic influence may cause these cells to proliferate and produce chronic lymphatic leukemia or lymphomas. B cells bind antigen and then divide to form plasma cells. The cells secrete an antibody product identical to that of the receptor on the B cell from which it was derived.

25. The answer is C (2, 4). *(Isselbacher, ed 9. pp 1567-1568. Stiehm, ed 2. p 620.)* Circulating immunoglobulins that can inactivate coagulation factors have been described in hemophilia, systemic lupus erythematosus (SLE), immediately postpartum, and in elderly people of both sexes. The antibody is usually IgG in nature, and in hemophilia the subclass IgG_4 has been incriminated. The antibody can inactivate many factors, but antibodies to factors VIII and X are the most common. In conditions other than SLE, immunosuppressive therapy has failed to affect significantly the levels and functions of these antibodies. Such antibodies should be monitored routinely in the presence of SLE.

26-29. The answers are: 26-B, 27-B, 28-C, 29-C. *(Bach, pp 320, 353, 665, 755. Isselbacher, ed 9. pp 306, 319, 333, 365-367.)* Contact sensitivity results from a delayed hypersensitivity immunologic reaction that occurs when the sensitizing agent forms a complex with a skin protein. A classic example of such sensitivity would be the reaction occurring following exposure to poison ivy. These delayed hypersensitivity reactions are mediated by thymus-derived T lymphocytes.

Allograft rejection can occur as the result of humoral immune reactions. Being thymus-dependent, however, these reactions are mediated by T lymphocytes. Although a graft being transplanted to a patient with preformed antibody can result in almost immediate rejection, such is not the usual way that grafts are rejected. More commonly, a chronic graft rejection occurs as a result of a classic cell-mediated immune reaction against the histocompatibility antigens present on the allograft; this is a clear example of a T-cell mediated reaction.

Arthus' reactions are immunologic responses that result when complement components are activated by immune complexes. The immune complexes usually involve IgG antibody complexed onto the antigen. The activation of the complement cascade results in the formation of biologically active complement components that can cause vasodilatation and attract polymorphonuclear leukocytes into the local tissue area. It is this polymorphonuclear mobilization that causes the typical Arthus' reaction, usually seen some four hours after antigen is introduced into the skin. The histologic features consist mainly of polymorphonuclear infiltration and some hemorrhage.

Monoclonal proliferation in multiple myeloma usually involves either the IgG or IgA class of antibody. IgM monoclonal proliferations in multiple myeloma have been described, but are much more common in Waldenstrom's macroglobulinemia. Presumably, this tendency for IgG and IgA proliferation would suggest that the more mature B-lymphocyte series that produces IgG and IgA is involved in the malignant disturbance.

30-32. The answers are: 30-B, 31-E, 32-A. *(Isselbacher, ed 9. p 547. Vyas, pp 22, 25, 72, 275.)* T-cell cytotoxicity frequently is measured in a number of experimental and clinical situations. Most frequently, this involves attempts to determine whether patients' T lymphocytes are capable of destroying their own or someone else's tumor cells. While morphologic examination of target cells is occasionally performed for this purpose, it is more objective and reproducible to use a target cell that is isotope-labeled. Radioactive isotopes of chromium have proved very valuable in this connection; chromium is rapidly taken into the lymphocyte, and although there is some spontaneous release, significant amounts of chromium will not be released until the cell has been killed. Thereupon, the addition of appropriate T cells enables a direct measurement in a gamma counter of the cytotoxicity induced by the added cells.

For routine quantitative immunoglobulin assays, simple techniques will suffice. Accuracy to within a few milligrams percent can be obtained by the gel diffusion technique. In gel diffusion, sera suspected of containing a given amount of immunoglobulin is placed in one well of an agar plate, while in a second well is deposited antisera known to contain antibody against a given immunoglobulin class. Through the agar, the antigen (in this case the suspected immunoglobulin) and the anti-immunoglobulin sera diffuse towards each other. A precipitin line occurs on contact, and from the degree of precipitation the quantity of antibody present can be determined.

IgE antibody is present in very small quantities in biologic fluids. Although biologically extremely potent even at these tiny concentrations, IgE antibody cannot be detected by routine gel diffusion. Thus, its quantitation requires radioimmunoassay using very sensitive antisera directed against IgE. The antisera is labeled with radioactive iodine and accuracy is excellent down to as little as 10 to 20 ng/ml.

33-35. The answers are: 33-A, 34-C, 35-B. *(Bach, p 303. Gell, ed 3. p 719. Isselbacher, ed 9. pp 279-280, 330, 1601. Stiehm, ed 2. p 8.)* IgA is an antibody that exists both in the serum and the mucosal surface. In the serum, IgA usually is in the form of a trimer that cannot diffuse into normal mucosal secretions and thus is useless in protecting mucosal areas. IgA produced by B lymphocytes within the intestinal lymphoid tissue is secreted by plasma cells in the form of a dimer. The steric form of this dimer molecule is such that it will enable physical interaction between the molecule and a substance produced by intestinal epithelial cells known as secretory piece.

Secretory piece combines with IgA and supplies an essential transport mechanism for the rapid movement of IgA to the mucosal surface from the depths of the intestinal crypts. Rare cases of normal IgA production but absent secretory piece have now been described. Secretory piece is strongly antigenic, and thus good antisera are available that allow a gel diffusion technique to quantitate the amount of secretory piece present in secretions.

Cyclophosphamide is an immunosuppressive drug with a number of side effects besides its cytotoxic effect on both B and T lymphocytes. The drug causes temporary loss of body hair; in the concentrated form in which it is secreted by the kidney, cyclophosphamide can cause a nasty hemorrhagic cystitis unless patients taking the drug drink fluids copiously. Such fluid intake usually averts cystitis. Cyclophosphamide exerts its major effect on B lymphocytes, although in large doses T lymphocytes are affected as well.

Germinal centers are areas in lymph nodes and in the spleen where B cells congregate. These areas are highly organized and so constructed that dendritic cells are capable of holding antigen (brought to these areas by lymphoid vessels) in a way that optimizes antigen recognition. In lymph nodes, these germinal centers cluster just underneath the capsule of the node and are surrounded by paracortical areas full of T lymphocytes. In the spleen, germinal centers cluster around the splenic vein. These anatomic aspects of germinal centers are important because, in examining lymph node and spleen specimens especially from patients afflicted with malignancy, alterations within these areas frequently suggest disturbances of B-cell function. Significantly, when B cells are involved in immunopathogenic mechanisms, such as in the synovium in rheumatoid arthritis, the aggregations of B cells tend to form germinal centers in these local areas.

36-39. The answers are: 36-C, 37-C, 38-C, 39-C. *(Isselbacher, ed 9. pp 1872-1873. Park, p 375.)* Rheumatoid factor usually is an IgM antibody that has activity against aggregated or altered IgG, although rheumatoid factors of all immunoglobulin classes have been described. Juvenile rheumatoid arthritis, for instance, not uncommonly exhibits IgG rheumatoid factors that have antibody activity against aggregated or altered IgG. Rheumatoid factors are thus autoantibodies, and it seems certain that the macromolecular complexes so formed can activate complement mechanisms and cause joint damage. The activation of the complement cascade results in polymorphonuclear leukocyte infiltration into the joint fluid with subsequent damage to synovial tissues.

Though most frequently found in adult rheumatoid arthritis (90 percent), rheumatoid factors are also found in juvenile rheumatoid arthritis (25 percent), Sjögren's syndrome (75 percent), systemic lupus erythematosus (30 percent), and occasionally other inflammatory diseases, including leprosy and infectious mononucleosis. It is possible that an infectious agent generates an aggregated or altered antibody to that agent, and that this changed immunoglobulin stimulates the production of the rheumatoid factor in a susceptible individual.

Rheumatoid arthritis can occur in agammaglobulinemic individuals, who by definition are incapable of making rheumatoid factors; it can also occur in a seronegative form in which no autoantibodies can be found. Usually such cases are milder than the seropositive cases of rheumatoid arthritis, but it raises the possibility that mechanisms other than the activation of complement by rheumatoid complexes may be important in the immunopathogenesis of rheumatoid arthritis.

Infectious Disease

DIRECTIONS: Each question below contains five suggested answers. Choose the **one best** response to each question.

40. All the following statements concerning herpes simplex encephalitis are true EXCEPT that

(A) it is a common form of nonepidemic adult encephalitis in the United States
(B) the causative virus can usually be isolated from cerebrospinal fluid
(C) the cerebrospinal fluid in affected patients often contains red blood cells during acute illness
(D) it may result in necrosis of brain tissue and high fatality
(E) evidence of a localized brain lesion may be found on electroencephalography

41. In a patient who has mitral valve insufficiency, prophylactic antibiotic treatment is recommended for all the following procedures EXCEPT

(A) cardiac catheterization
(B) prostatectomy
(C) cystoscopy
(D) sigmoidoscopy
(E) endoscopy

42. A 20-year-old man is admitted to the hospital with a four-day history of fever, chills, nonproductive cough, and earache. The most likely cause of his infection is

(A) *Mycobacterium tuberculosis*
(B) *Mycoplasma pneumoniae*
(C) *Klebsiella pneumoniae*
(D) *Diplococcus pneumoniae*
(E) type A influenza

43. A 60-year-old man had lived in Mexico for approximately six months. A year later he is seen for pyrexia, weight loss, and right upper quadrant pain. His oral cholecystogram is normal and liver function tests are mildly, but not diagnostically, abnormal. Which of the following would be the most useful diagnostic procedure?

(A) Serologic tests for amebiasis
(B) Examination of the stool for ova and parasites
(C) Examination of fluid aspirated from the liver
(D) A diagnostic trial of chloroquine
(E) A diagnostic trial of metronidazole

44. In treating a 24-year-old woman for infectious syphilis in the last trimester of pregnancy, the LEAST appropriate antibiotic regimen would be

(A) cephaloridine, 0.5 g daily for 10 days
(B) erythromycin, 2 g daily for 14 days
(C) tetracycline, 2 g daily for 10 days
(D) intramuscular penicillin G benzathine, 2.4 million units
(E) penicillin G procaine, 600,000 units daily for ten days

45. *Pseudomonas aeruginosa* is a gram-negative motile rod that is responsible for much serious illness. Which of the following statements about infection with this organism is true?

(A) It may result in a bacteremia that carries a 45 percent mortality rate
(B) It may produce ecthyma gangrenosum in the damaged skin of burn victims
(C) It may require the use of *Pseudomonas* hyperimmune globulin if the organism does not respond quickly to antibiotics
(D) It may result in an endocarditis that metastasizes to joints and adrenal glands if the patient has had prior valvular disease
(E) It may produce pulmonary infections that are characterized by the presence of microabscesses

46. Which of the following antibiotics is inactive against anaerobic bacteria?

(A) Penicillin
(B) Clindamycin
(C) Metronidazole
(D) Gentamicin
(E) Carbenicillin

47. Chagas' disease exhibits all the following findings EXCEPT

(A) esophageal dilatation
(B) megacolon
(C) pancreatic pseudocysts
(D) unilateral conjunctivitis with edema of eyelids and face
(E) subacute myocarditis

48. Calcified cysts occurring in either liver or lung, often many years after initial infection with the responsible organism, are characteristic of which of the following diseases?

(A) Fascioliasis
(B) Amebiasis
(C) Giardiasis
(D) Hydatid disease
(E) Intestinal bilharziasis

49. Appropriate specimens for attempted virus isolation or recognition differ with particular viruses. All the following viruses may be isolated from the sources specified EXCEPT

(A) echoviruses from stool or rectal swab
(B) rubella from urine
(C) varicella-zoster from vesicular fluid
(D) cytomegalovirus from throat swab
(E) arboviruses from cerebrospinal fluid

50. Pinworm infection is characterized by which of the following observations?

(A) It is usually diagnosed on stool examination by identifying infective larvae of *Enterobius vermicularis*
(B) It can be diagnosed by finding eggs in the duodenal mucosa
(C) It often results in severe pruritus ani
(D) It can be eradicated fron a household by treating the family member having the most severe symptoms
(E) It is usually confined to a single member of a family

51. A fresh-water swimmer develops macules on his lower extremities ten hours after bathing in an area known to harbor cercariae of duck schistosomes. The natural history of this "swimmer's itch" includes

(A) the development of microscopic hematuria in about two months
(B) the development of a self-limited dermatitis
(C) the late development of cirrhosis and splenomegaly
(D) rapid abatement of fever after treatment with topical thiabendazole
(E) human-to-human transmission to persons in close physical contact

52. Infection by *Plasmodium falciparum* (clinical falciparum malaria in humans) is associated with all the following clinical signs or syndromes EXCEPT

(A) blackwater fever (hemoglobinuric fever)
(B) resistance to 4-aminoquinoline drugs such as chloroquine
(C) febrile episodes occurring every 72 hours
(D) cerebral malaria with coma
(E) high density parasitemia

53. All the following statements concerning maculopapular rashes associated with infectious diseases are true EXCEPT that

(A) *Mycoplasma* infections cause a maculopapular rash characterized by a prominent palmar or plantar involvement
(B) erythema infectiosum (fifth disease) is associated with a confluent erythema over the cheeks and symmetric eruptions on the trunk, arms, and legs but rarely on the palms and soles
(C) echoviruses cause a maculopapular rash that may be associated with petechiae
(D) exanthem subitum (roseola infantum) produces a mild maculopapular rash that is largely asymptomatic even though it lasts five to ten days
(E) maculopapular rashes are common in typhoid fever

54. A 32-year-old woman presents at an emergency room with a three-day history of severe headache associated with photophobia, drowsiness, and some confusion. She also complains of some arthralgia and loss of appetite. Physical examination reveals only minimal signs of meningeal irritation. Her temperature is 38.4°C (101°F). Cerebrospinal fluid findings consist of a mononuclear pleocytosis, a small increase in protein, normal glucose levels, and the absence of demonstrable microorganisms. Of the following, which is the most likely diagnosis?

(A) Lymphocytic choriomeningitis
(B) Aseptic meningitis caused by an echovirus
(C) Aseptic meningitis caused by a herpesvirus
(D) Infectious mononucleosis
(E) Behçet's disease

55. All the following disorders or syndromes are attributable to toxoplasmosis EXCEPT

(A) a syndrome simulating mononucleosis
(B) hydrocephalus, microcephaly, and cerebral calcifications
(C) recrudescence in immunocompromised patients
(D) focal chorioretinitis
(E) gastroenteritis

56. Rabies, an acute viral disease of the mammalian central nervous system, is transmitted by infective secretions (usually saliva). Which of the following statements about this disease is the most accurate?

(A) The disease is caused by a reovirus that elicits both complement fixing and hemagglutinating antibodies useful in the diagnosis of the disease
(B) The incubation period is variable and, although ten days is the most common elapsed time between infection and symptoms, some cases remain asymptomatic for 30 days
(C) Only 30 percent of infected patients will survive
(D) In the United States, the skunk and the bat have been the most important recent sources of human disease
(E) Wild animals that have bitten and are suspected of being rabid should be killed and their brains examined for virus particles by electron microscopy

57. Two days before the end of a two-week vacation in the Caribbean, a 43-year-old man who had always enjoyed good health experiences nausea, flatulence, epigastric discomfort, and watery diarrhea. Three weeks later, the diarrhea having persisted unabated, he consults his physician for what he believes to be a case of "traveler's diarrhea." The only abnormality found on stool examination is the presence of the trophozoite stages of *Giardia lamblia*. All the following statements concerning this patient's disorder are true EXCEPT that

(A) radiography may reveal irritability of the duodenal bulb
(B) it is important to check the stools of the patient's sexual partner for the same protozoan
(C) the significance of the stool finding is not clear; 3.8 percent of all stools examined in the United States reveals *Giardia lamblia*
(D) IgA deficiency, although commonly associated with *Giardia lamblia* infestation, is unlikely to be a factor in this case
(E) rapid weight loss associated with the diarrhea would be consistent with a diagnosis of giardiasis

58. A 22-year-old man who has just returned from Southeast Asia has a purulent urethral discharge. A Gram stain of the discharge showed many polymorphonuclear leukocytes containing gram-negative diplococci. The patient was treated with oral probenecid, 1 g, and intramuscular penicillin G procaine, 4.8 million units. His symptoms persisted, and he was treated again with the same regimen without improvement. The next step in the management of this patient would be to

(A) culture the urethral discharge on Thayer-Martin agar plates
(B) request antibiotic sensitivities on the organism
(C) treat him with intramuscular penicillin G benzathine (Bicillin)
(D) treat him with intramuscular spectinomycin
(E) do none of the above

DIRECTIONS: Each question below contains four suggested answers of which **one** or **more** is correct. Choose the answer:

A	if	**1, 2, and 3**	are correct
B	if	**1 and 3**	are correct
C	if	**2 and 4**	are correct
D	if	**4**	is correct
E	if	**1, 2, 3, and 4**	are correct

59. A patient who has alcoholic cirrhosis that is moderately well controlled presents with increasing ascites, abdominal pain, and a deteriorating mental status. His temperature is 38.4° (101°F), rectally. Bowel sounds are hypoactive. As part of the evaluation of his pyrexia, peritoneal fluid is obtained. The fluid is cloudy and the white blood cell count is $400/mm^3$, 80 percent of which are polymorphonuclear forms. Ascitic fluid protein is 2 g/100 ml. Gram stain of the fluid is negative. The physician should initiate which of the following steps?

(1) Start the patient on clindamycin
(2) Start the patient on gentamicin
(3) Treat the patient for impending hepatic coma
(4) Perform an exploratory laparotomy

60. Whipworm infection or trichuriasis is characterized by which of the following observations?

(1) It is found in the southeastern United States
(2) It commonly causes no symptoms
(3) It may cause rectal prolapse
(4) It is diagnosed by duodenal aspiration

61. *Streptococcus (Diplococcus) pneumoniae* is still responsible for a significant number of deaths. A vaccine containing capsular polysaccharides from the 14 pneumococcal types responsible for 80 percent of pneumococcal infections in the United States is now available. Patients who should receive this vaccine include

(1) children who experience, in the first year of life, three attacks of otitis media caused by the pneumococcus
(2) patients with functional or anatomic asplenia
(3) patients with sickle-cell disease who have not received a booster dose of vaccine for two years
(4) patients over 55 years of age who have chronic-cardiovascular disease

62. The central nervous system may be involved in infectious diseases caused by which of the following pathogens?

(1) *Nocardia asteroides*
(2) *Cryptococcus neoformans*
(3) *Mucor*
(4) *Coccidioides immitis*

SUMMARY OF DIRECTIONS

A	B	C	D	E
1, 2, 3 only	1, 3 only	2, 4 only	4 only	All are correct

63. A 60-year-old man complains of symptoms that are compatible with an acute urinary tract infection. This episode is the third such infection in 12 months. The urine culture is positive for *Escherichia coli.* A diagnosis of chronic bacterial prostatitis may be strengthened on the basis of which of the following procedures?

(1) Intravenous pyelography
(2) Physical examination
(3) Urinalysis
(4) Quantitative culture of split urine samples

64. The transmission of trichinosis to humans is effectively controlled by

(1) cooking fresh pork to a temperature of at least 65.6°C (150°F), or until it turns from pink to white
(2) regular inspection of pork products for the presence of cysts
(3) maintaining pork at a temperature of −27°C (−16°F) for at least 36 hours before cooking
(4) adequate cooking of garbage that is fed to hogs

65. A 28-year-old woman is brought to an emergency room with an infection in a foot wound sustained 7 days earlier. Examination reveals a moderate degree of cellulitis associated with the wound, diplopia, dysphonia, and weakness. Primary immunization at four years of age had consisted of three doses of tetanus toxoid and one booster 8 years later. She should now be treated with

(1) wound debridement
(2) trivalent botulinal antitoxin
(3) tetanus toxoid
(4) hyperimmune antitetanus gamma globulin

66. *Histoplasma capsulatum* may be associated with which of the following conditions?

(1) Pneumonia
(2) Pulmonary cavities
(3) Meningitis
(4) Febrile hepatosplenomegaly

67. A lifelong resident of Connecticut traveled to Arizona to work on a water project in the desert. Shortly after beginning work he developed fever, cough, and shortness of breath. Other findings that he might be expected to develop include

(1) erythema nodosum
(2) arthralgias
(3) pneumonia
(4) a fleeting macular rash

68. Which of the following statements about primary subacute pyogenic osteomyelitis are true?

(1) It often affects the frontal bone over the frontal sinus
(2) It usually is caused by staphylococci
(3) It often is associated with disease of the paranasal sinuses
(4) It often affects the metaphysis of long bones

69. A 25-year-old woman who has systemic lupus erythematosus becomes pregnant. Her VDRL test is positive. Previous tests for syphilis on the patient are unavailable. Blood is drawn for a fluorescent treponemal antibody absorption (FTA-ABS) test. Correct statements concerning the interpretation of this test include which of the following?

(1) If FTA-ABS negative, the patient does not have syphilis
(2) If FTA-ABS positive, the *Treponema pallidum* immobilization (TPI) test may be positive
(3) If FTA-ABS positive, the TPI test may be negative
(4) If FTA-ABS positive, the patient has syphilis

70. Bacterial meningitis in the neonatal infant frequently is caused by which of the following organisms?

(1) *Streptococcus (Diplococcus) pneumoniae*
(2) Group B *Streptococcus*
(3) *Hemophilus influenzae*
(4) *Escherichia coli*

71. Lethal, necrotizing bronchopneumonia occurring during epidemics of influenza A or B appears to be characteristic of infection with which of the following organisms?

(1) *Mycoplasma*
(2) *Klebsiella pneumoniae*
(3) Group A beta-hemolytic *Streptococcus*
(4) *Staphylococcus aureus*

72. A 68-year-old man with a history of bronchiectasis is admitted to the hospital with severe headache, aphasia, and right arm weakness of one days duration. The presumptive diagnosis is a brain abscess. This diagnosis is compatible with which of the following results?

(1) Negative cerebrospinal fluid culture
(2) An abnormal electroencephalogram
(3) A normal carotid arteriogram
(4) An abnormal brain scan

73. A diabetic patient who requires insulin is seen in the emergency room with a painfully swollen eye, proptosis, and loss of external eye movements. She is acidotic; tenderness is elicited over the frontal sinus of the affected side. Rapid involvement of the other eye would suggest which of the following disorders?

(1) Osteomyelitis
(2) Orbital cellulitis
(3) Mucormycosis
(4) Cavernous sinus thrombosis

SUMMARY OF DIRECTIONS

A	B	C	D	E
1, 2, 3 only	1, 3 only	2, 4 only	4 only	All are correct

74. A ten-year-old Puerto Rican youth who has recently immigrated has his stool examined at a clinic in New York. Viable eggs of *Schistosoma mansoni* are present. Which of the following statements concerning this youngster are correct?

(1) A rectal biopsy should be performed to confirm the presence of viable eggs in the mucosa before starting treatment
(2) The presence of viable eggs means that the patient is infectious and can directly transmit the disease
(3) The patient is a public health hazard while in New York
(4) Niridazole is an effective agent in children of this age

75. Correct statements regarding herpes zoster (shingles) include which of the following?

(1) It probably results from the reactivation of latent infection in persons who previously have had chickenpox
(2) It usually causes a bilateral skin eruption in a dermatomal distribution
(3) It is often associated with depression of delayed hypersensitivity by immunosuppressive chemotherapy
(4) Severe pain in an affected dermatome usually precedes the onset of the vesicular lesions and lasts until the skin manifestations clear

76. A 20-year-old man is admitted to the hospital; his chest x-rays are shown below. He is producing copious amounts of sputum and appears moderately ill; his oral temperature is 38.4°C (101°F). He reports that he has lost approximately 10 pounds in the past two months and complains of drenching night sweats during that period. Which of the following findings would be expected in this patient at this time?

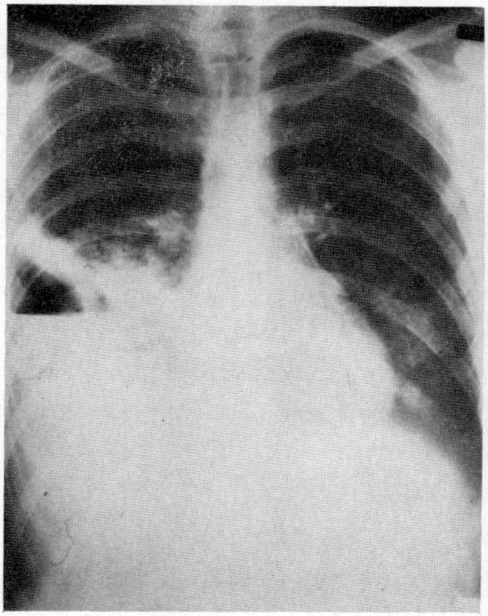

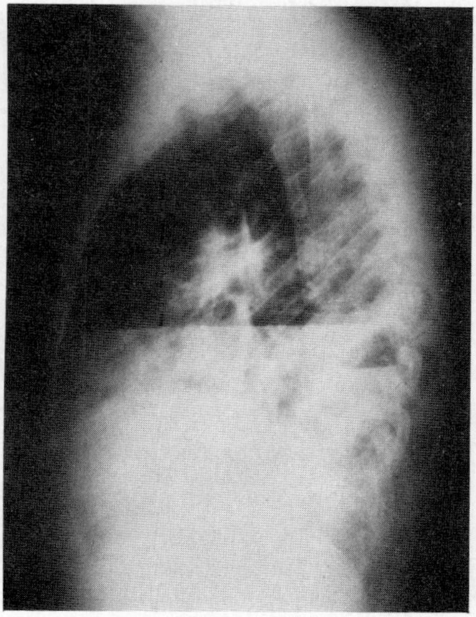

(1) Mixed gram-positive and gram-negative organisms in the sputum
(2) An absent gag reflex
(3) A history of drug abuse, alcohol abuse, or both
(4) A positive tuberculin test

DIRECTIONS: The groups of questions below consist of lettered choices followed by several numbered items. For each numbered item select the **one** lettered choice with which it is **most** closely associated. Each lettered choice may be used once, more than once, or not at all.

Questions 77-81

Match the following.

(A) Cephalothin
(B) Cephaloridine
(C) Cefazolin
(D) Cephalexin
(E) None of the above

77. Has marked activity against enterococci

78. Is highly effective in treating staphylococcal meningitis

79. Is the most resistant of the cephalosporins to hydrolysis by staphylococcal beta-lactamases

80. Its major advantages over other cephalosporins are the higher blood levels attained and the lower incidence of pain after intramuscular administration

81. Is the most consistent of the cephalosporins in attaining therapeutic levels in the bile

Questions 82-85

For each description that follows, select the disorder with which it is most likely to be associated.

(A) Renal cortex abscess
(B) Renal medulla abscess
(C) Perinephric abscess
(D) Ureteral stone
(E) Renal tuberculosis

82. It almost always follows hematogenous seeding from a bacteremia

83. The urine of affected patients is usually sterile and without pyuria or hematuria

84. Gram-negative organisms are commonly seen on stain of the urinary sediment from affected patients

85. The characteristic organism responsible is *Staphylococcus aureus*

Questions 86-90

For each description of a fungal infection that follows, select the microorganism with which it is most closely associated.

(A) *Blastomyces dermatitidis*
(B) *Histoplasma capsulatum*
(C) *Coccidioides immitis*
(D) *Aspergillus fumigatus*
(E) *Cryptococcus neoformans*

86. Disease occurs sporadically throughout the world. Susceptibility is increased by exogenous corticosteroids and in patients afflicted with lymphoma. Microorganism is isolated from pigeon droppings

87. Disease may be transmitted via fomites outside of endemic areas. Microorganism is isolated from soil especially around rodent burrows and is highly infectious

88. Disease associated with demolition of old buildings and excavations in endemic areas. Microorganism is isolated from soil high in organic content, especially bird droppings

89. Susceptibility to disease increases in patients who have quantitative or qualitative granulocyte defects or who are receiving corticosteroids. Saprophytic endobronchial—as well as invasive—infection occurs. Microorganism is isolated from decaying vetetation

90. Disease restricted to southeastern United States. Cutaneous, pulmonary, and disseminated forms may occur

Questions 91-95

For each antibiotic that follows, select the side effect with which it is most closely associated.

(A) Vestibular toxicity
(B) Ototoxicity
(C) Decreased protein synthesis
(D) Photosensitivity
(E) Liver toxicity

91. Chloramphenicol

92. Demeclocycline (Declomycin)

93. Minocycline

94. Rifampin

95. Vancomycin

Questions 96-99

For each complication of infection that follows, select the causative organism with which it is most likely to be associated.

(A) *Neisseria meningitides*
(B) *Hemophilus influenzae*
(C) *Brucella melitensis*
(D) *Clostridium perfringens*
(E) *Mycobacterium leprae*

96. Depression or psychoneuroses

97. Chronic sinusitis

98. Herpes labialis

99. Hemolytic anemia

Questions 100-104

For each description of a patient that follows, select the x-ray (shown on this and the succeeding two pages) with which it is most likely to be associated.

100. A 40-year-old alcoholic man is admitted to the hospital with a two-week history of fever, cough, and hemoptysis. Sputum culture is positive for *Staphylococcus aureus.* He is being treated with cephalothin but there is no response

101. A 20-year-old man afflicted with Hodgkin's disease is admitted to the hospital complaining of five days of increasingly severe vesicular rash and shortness of breath of one days duration

102. A 58-year-old male outpatient has a one-year history of cough and intermittent hemoptysis. Sputum cultures are positive for *Aspergillus fumigatus*

103. A 48-year-old man is seen in the outpatient department for evaluation of shortness of breath and wheezing. Sputum culture is positive for *A. fumigatus.* Skin and serologic tests for aspergillosis are positive as well

104. A 48-year-old woman who is receiving intensive treatment for thrombotic thrombocytopenic purpura is admitted to the hospital with fever, productive cough, and left-sided weakness

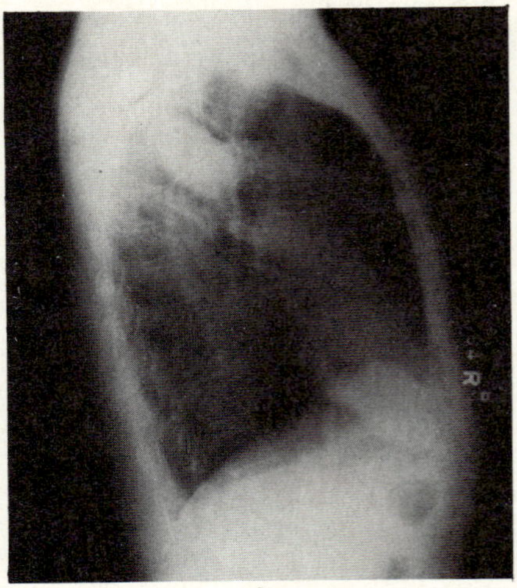

A_1

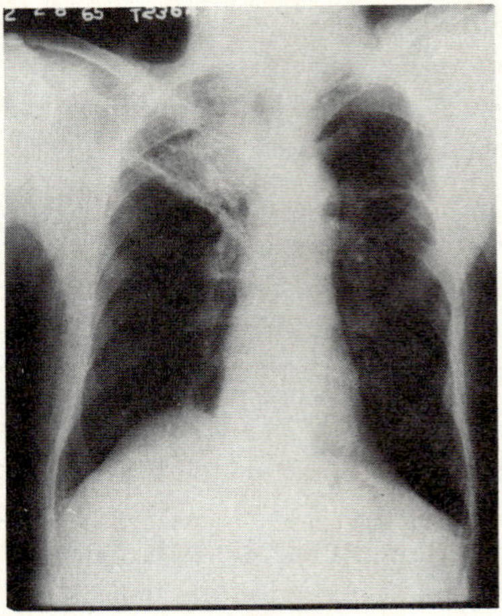

A_2

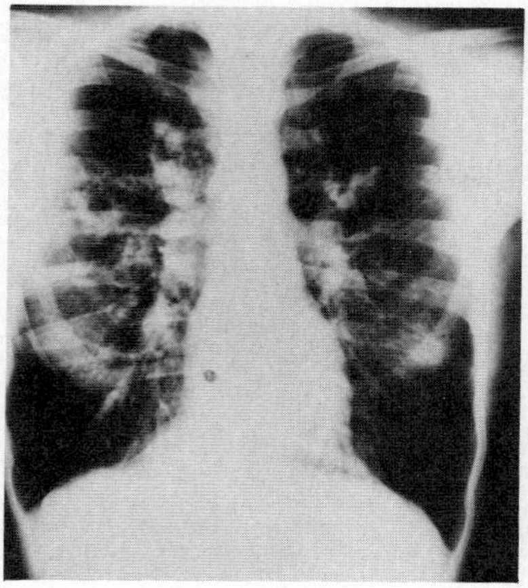

B$_1$

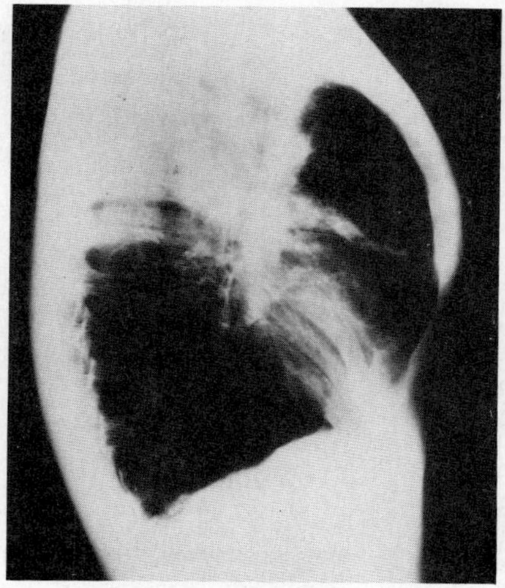

B$_2$

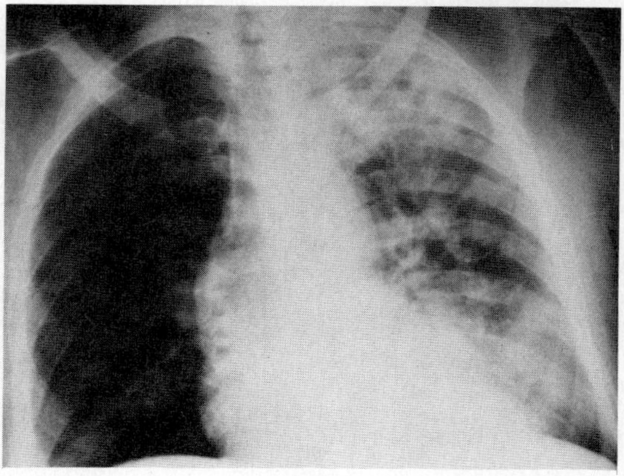

C

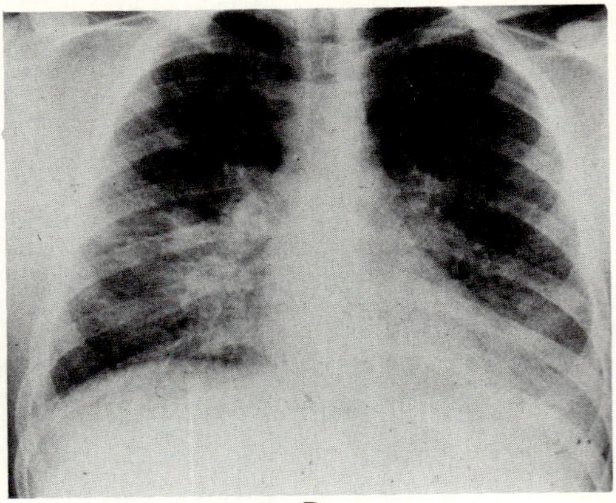

D

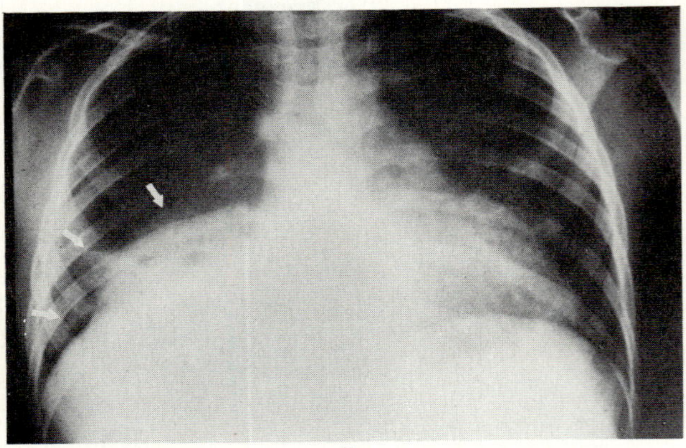

E_1

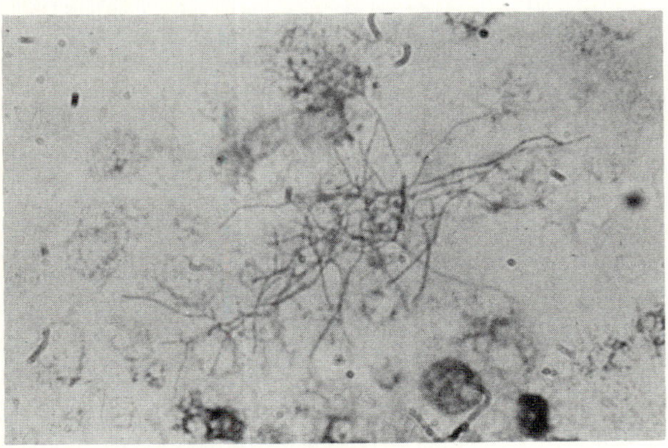

E_2

Questions 105-109

For each pair of drugs that follows, select the type of drug interaction with which the pair is most likely to be associated.

(A) Enhanced anticoagulant effect
(B) Enhanced nephrotoxicity
(C) Increased incidence of thrombocytopenia
(D) Increased incidence of bone marrow suppression
(E) No significant toxicity

105. Tetracycline and dicumarol

106. Chloramphenicol and dicumarol

107. Azathioprine and allopurinol

108. Trimethoprim and thiazides

109. Carbenicillin and gentamicin

Questions 110-112

For each phrase that follows, select the drug combination with which it is most likely to be associated.

(A) Chloramphenicol and phenytoin (Dilantin)
(B) Isoniazid and rifampin
(C) Tetracycline and antacids
(D) Erythromycin and calcium supplements
(E) Isoniazid and ethambutol

110. Decreased absorption of one drug due to the effect of the other

111. Increased risk of hepatotoxicity

112. Prolonged half-life of one drug due to a shared metabolic pathway with the other

Questions 113-117

For each description of food poisoning that follows, select the microorganism with which it is most closely associated.

(A) *Clostridium perfringens*
(B) *Staphylococcus aureus*
(C) *Shigella sonnei*
(D) *Vibrio parahaemolyticus*
(E) *Yersinia enterocolitica*

113. Severe cramps, diarrhea, and occasional nausea and vomiting. Associated with cold or reheated cooked meats, gravy, or stews

114. Severe cramps, bloody diarrhea, and fever. Epidemics associated with contaminated water and food have been reported

115. Moderate to severe cramps, bloody diarrhea, and fever. Epidemics in the United States have been associated with ingestion of contaminated crabs

116. Severe nausea, vomiting, and occasional cramps and diarrhea. Associated with contaminated meats and dairy products

117. Severe abdominal pain and tenderness that may mimic appendicitis. Recent outbreaks in the United States have been associated with contaminated water

Infectious Disease Answers

40. The answer is B. *(Hammon, DM February:31-35, 1973. Isselbacher, ed 9. pp 848-849.)* In active cases of herpes simplex encephalitis, it is rare to culture herpesvirus from the cerebrospinal fluid. Once found, the virus is easily grown; a biopsy specimen from an affected part of the brain, procured early in the course of the disease, is the best means of isolating it. The isolation of the virus may in the future dictate therapy with an agent such as adenine arabinoside.

41. The answer is A. *(Isselbacher, ed 9. pp 1100-1103. Kaye, p 251.)* Although no evidence exists that prophylactic antibiotic therapy prevents endocarditis, prophylaxis is recommended for all procedures that may generate bacteremias. Following cardiac catheterization, blood cultures obtained from a distal vein rarely are positive. Thus, prophylactic antibiosis is not currently recommended for cardiac catheterization. Bacteremia occurs commonly following other procedures such as endoscopy, cystoscopy, sigmoidoscopy, and prostate surgery.

42. The answer is B. *(Isselbacher, ed 9. pp 759-761, 1537. Youmans, pp 271-291.)* Viral or mycoplasmal pneumonias characteristically have a subacute onset and produce low grade fever, nonproductive cough, and chills, but not rigor. Bullous myringitis causes earaches in as many as one-fourth of adolescent and college age patients afflicted with *Mycoplasma pneumoniae* infections, and is the clue to the diagnosis in the case presented in the question. Pneumococcal pneumonia is characterized by a sudden onset of high fever, rigors and a productive cough with purulent or bloody sputum. In viral or mycoplasmal pneumonia the inflammation is interstitial and produces a diffuse infiltrate on x-ray; the inflammation of pneumococcal pneumonia, however, involves the alveoli and small airways leading to an accumulation of fluid in these areas and consolidation on x-ray. A diagnosis of mycoplasmal pneumonia may be confirmed by demonstrating a significant increase in cold agglutinins or complement-fixing mycoplasmal antibody. Rarely, hemolytic anemia occurs from two to three weeks after the onset of symptoms. It is associated with cold agglutination titers greater than 1:500, although it may occur with lower titers. The hemolytic anemia is transient and coincides with clinical recovery.

43. The answer is D. *(Barbour, Am J Med 53:331, 1972. Isselbacher, ed 9. pp 863-867.)* Amebiasis is prevalent in tropical and subtropical climates. Serologic tests, among them indirect hemagglutination, complement fixation, and agar gel diffusion, are positive in 80 to 100 percent of patients who have hepatic amebiasis. Response to chloroquine, measured by rapid decrease in both symptoms and abscess size, is the most important diagnostic test for this disorder. While metronidazole is an effective agent against trophozoites at all sites, a positive clinical response to it would not be diagnostic for amebic abscess because it also inhibits anaerobic bacteria. The classic anchovy-paste color associated with fluid aspirated from an abscess is by no means diagnostic of hepatic amebiasis. Barbour and Juniper found such fluid in only 2 of 16 initial aspirates from amebic abscesses.

44. The answer is C. *(Burrow, pp 397-399. Isselbacher, ed 9. p 720.)* Syphilis in pregnancy is a serious disease that may result in late abortion, stillbirth, or a congenitally infected infant. The drug of choice in the therapy of all forms of syphilis is penicillin. Various regimens employing penicillin G benzathine or penicillin G procaine are acceptable. Relatively safe alternatives to penicillin in pregnancy include cephaloridine and erythromycin. Tetracycline, although effective against syphilis, should be avoided in pregnancy because the drug is deposited in fetal teeth and bones and may cause maternal hepatotoxicity.

45. The answer is E. *(Isselbacher, ed 9. pp 634-636.)* Infection with *Pseudomonas aeruginosa* most frequently occurs in the hospital environment, the organism being acquired from sources other than the patient's normal flora. Bacteremia is an especially serious complication of infection that is associated with a mortality prognosis of 75 percent. Such bacteremia is clinically indistinguishable from blood stream infections with other bacterial species, except that it may be associated with a skin lesion—echthymic gangrenosum—best described as a round indurated purple-to-black area about 1 cm in diameter with an ulcerated center surrounded by a zone of erythema. These lesions can occur in any patient infected with the organism. Rarely, bacteremia is associated with the passing of green urine from the excretion of large amounts of hemoglobin pigment. Antibiotics are essential, though often unsuccessful in the management of established infection. As a prophylactic measure, hyperimmune gamma globulin has been found useful in patients with severe burns and cancer patients about to commence chemotherapy. It does not, as yet, have an established role in the management of ongoing infection. *Pseudomonas* infections may be associated with an endocarditis and, in a number of burn patients and drug addicts, the endocarditis has been found on normal heart valves. Pulmonary infection is characterized by the presence of microabscesses.

46. The answer is D. *(Finegold, J Infect Dis 124 suppl:56-58, 1971. Isselbacher, ed 9. pp 695-699.)* Most obligate anaerobic bacteria are highly resistant to gentamicin and other aminoglycosides. This is an important consideration in the design of therapeutic regimens for infections involving anaerobic bacteria, such as abdominal sepsis. Where gentamicin-sensitive organisms are implicated as well as anaerobic bacteria like *Bacteroides fragilis,* which may be penicillin-resistant, it is advisable to combine gentamicin with a drug such as clindamycin or carbenicillin to assure the required antibiotic coverage.

47. The answer is C. *(Hunter, ed 5. pp 440-449. Isselbacher, ed 9. pp 876-879.)* Chagas' disease, caused by protozoa of the genus *Trypanosoma*, involves the development of both megaesophagus and megacolon as a consequence of neuronal damage. The unilateral oculoglandular complex known as Romaña's sign and myocarditis are also well recognized features of the disease.

48. The answer is D. *(Hunter, ed 5. pp 609-615. Isselbacher, ed 9. pp 917-918.)* Hydatid cysts of the liver are known to survive for as long as fifty years after infested patients have left an epidemic region. Ruptured cysts can produce severe allergic reactions; bacterial superinfection of cysts can result in abscesses; and bone cysts can generate pathologic fractures. Surgical removal, marsupialization, freezing, and the instillation of toxic materials such as formalin are current forms of treatment for hydatid hepatic cysts.

49. The answer is D. *(Isselbacher, ed 9. p 776.)* Cytomegalovirus infection will produce a clinical syndrome indistinguishable from infectious mononucleosis. However, differential diagnosis can be made by isolating the virus from the urine and often from the buffy coat of blood. Rubella viruses are isolated from the throat and the urine, while arboviruses can be isolated only from the cerebrospinal fluid or a piece of brain tissue. Echoviruses may be isolated from the throat, cerebrospinal fluid, and vesicular fluid but rarely from the urine. Herpes zoster can be isolated from vesicular fluid and occasionally from the lungs and myocardium of infected individuals.

50. The answer is C. *(Isselbacher, ed 9. p 899.)* Pruritus ani or vulvovaginitis are a part of the clinical symptomatology of pinworm infections. The eggs of *Enterobius vermicularis* are hardy at room temperature, and infection easily spreads throughout a household, particularly in a crowded environment. Hence, treatment of all members of the household and cleaning of the living area are required to prevent reinfection. Eggs of this parasite have been found in a 100,000-year-old coprolith, making it the oldest demonstrated infection of humans. Thirty to forty million persons in the United States and Canada are thought to carry this worm. Searching for ova in the feces is rarely helpful, but scrapings from under the nails may reveal ova. The usual location of the worms is the cecum, appendix, and adjacent large intestine. Thus, ova will not be found in the duodenal mucosa. Gravid females migrate through the anal canal, emerge partially or completely, and deposit eggs on the perianal skin. The preferred method of diagnosis is to press sticky cellophane tape firmly against the perianal area and then spread the preparation on a glass slide and examine it for ova under the lower power of a microscope.

51. The answer is B. *(Hunter, ed 5. pp 565-567. Isselbacher, ed 9. p 911.)* Human infection by the cercariae of one of the many nonhuman schistosomes is self-limited. On initial exposure, a mild dermatitis may not even be noticed. Sensitized persons develop more intense reactions, but the infection stops at this point without further progression. The disease is commonly found in Canada and the northern United States.

52. The answer is C. *(Hunter, ed 5. pp 353-396. Isselbacher, ed 9. p 870.)* The occurrence of fever every 72 hours is characteristic of early infection with *Plasmodium malariae*, or quartan malaria. This type of malaria can persist for many years with relapses as long as 20 years after infection. In falciparum malaria, however, a 48-hour cycle is seen.

53. The answer is D. *(Isselbacher, ed 9. pp 797-798.)* Enteroviruses such as echovirus can cause maculopapular rashes and occasionally papulovesicular or petechial rashes. Other viruses are capable of provoking erythema multiforme-like eruptions. The location of the rash provides a useful diagnostic criterion. Maculopapular rashes, in which there is a relative sparing of the palms and soles, are generally caused by viruses. Eruptions associated with drug reactions, bacteria, Mycoplasma, and Rickettsia often feature a prominent palmar and plantar eruption. The maculopapular rash of roseola is usually transient, lasting only a few hours and rarely as long as two days.

54. The answer is B. *(Isselbacher, ed 9. p 1967.)* The diagnosis of aseptic meningitis is suggested by (1) fever, (2) mild to moderately severe signs of meningeal irritation, (3) an accumulation of mononuclear and, more particularly, lymphocytic cells in the cerebrospinal fluid, and (4) an absence of the usual findings that indicate bacterial infection. The most frequent and severe symptom is headache associated with a morbidity that is not usually found in other febrile states. Although many infective agents have been incriminated in this condition, it is usually a virus that causes aseptic meningitis. Coxsackievirus, echovirus, mumps, and lymphocytic choriomeningitis account for 95 percent of confirmed cases of aseptic meningitis; coxsackie and echoviruses alone account for nearly 80 percent of cases. However, in as many as 25 percent of patients with aseptic meningitis there will be no microorganisms isolated from the cerebrospinal fluid. Infectious mononucleosis, influenza, leptospirosis, and rarely, herpes infections all can cause an aseptic meningitis. Behçet's disease is a rare affliction characterized by aseptic meningitis associated with uveitis, arthralgias, sterile skin abscesses following trauma, and thrombophlebitis.

55. The answer is E. *(Hunter, ed 5. pp 397-403. Isselbacher, ed 9. pp 879-885.)* In addition to those listed in the question, manifestations of toxoplasmosis include pericarditis, myocarditis, and pneumonitis but not gastroenteritis. Often there is a maculopapular, erythematous rash that characteristically does not involve the hands or feet.

56. The answer is D. *(Isselbacher, ed 9. pp 818-821.)* Rabies is caused by a bullet-shaped rhabdovirus. The presence of neutralizing antibody to a knob-like projection on the virus can be useful in diagnosis; a four-fold rise in the neutralizing antibody in serial serum samples is diagnostic in nonimmunized individuals. In the United States, dogs seldom are rabid. The animals that represent the most danger are wild skunks and bats; raccoons and foxes also are possible carriers. The incubation period is variable, ranging from 10 days to one year with a mean of one to two months. In humans, only three definite recoveries from established infection have been reported. Nonimmunized animals that have bitten should be killed and their brains examined for virus by immunofluorescent antibody staining. A negative fluorescent test removes the need to treat the bite victim, either actively or passively.

57. The answer is C. *(Isselbacher, ed 9. pp 887-888.)* *Giardia lamblia* is a pear-shaped multiflagellated protozoan that parasitizes the human small intestine. The organism is transmitted by the fecal-oral route. The infection is found worldwide, especially in regions of poor sanitation and personal hygiene. *Giardia lamblia* is diagnosed in 3.8 percent of examined stools in the United States and is the most frequently identified intestinal parasite. However, the finding of *Giardia lamblia* in the stool from the patient described in the question is highly significant. The organisms frequently cause "traveler's diarrhea," characteristically beginning late in the course of the travels and persisting for several weeks. Giardiasis is commonly associated with IgA deficiency, although IgA deficiency is not likely to be a factor in a previously well patient. Other conditions that predispose to giardiasis include gastrectomy and chronic pancreatitis. Irritability of the duodenal bulb often can be demonstrated radiographically. Rapid weight loss, along with lactase and dissacharidase deficiencies and general malabsorption, are commonly associated with giardiasis. A study in New York demonstrated that all male "nontravelers" who have this infection were homosexual. Even in asymptomatic sexual partners of giardiasis victims, it is important that the infection be ruled out as a precaution against dissemination of the disease.

58. The answer is D. *(Isselbacher, ed 9. p 627.)* Persistence of intracellular gram-negative diplococci in the urethral discharge of a patient being treated for gonococcal urethritis may suggest that the treatment has failed because of relatively drug-resistant gonococci rather than because of the presence of nonspecific urethritis. Recently, the highest incidence of penicillin-resistant gonococcal urethritis has been reported in Southeast Asia and on the west coast of the United States. The drug of choice in this situation is spectinomycin, which is resistant to the beta-lactamase elaborated by these otherwise resistant strains. Very large doses of penicillin might eradicate these infections but cannot be given intramuscularly. Penicillin G benzathine (Bicillin), effective in syphilis, is ineffective against gonococcal urethritis because the antibiotic does not achieve the peak levels required for cure.

59. The answer is A (1, 2, 3). *(Conn, Gastroenterology 70:455-457, 1976. Conn, Medicine 50:161-197, 1971. Isselbacher, ed 9. p 1482.)* Although dispute persists regarding the number of white blood cells and the percent granulocytes that can be considered normal in ascitic fluid, 300 or more white cells/mm^3, of which more than 25 percent are polymorphonuclear forms, is assumed to herald infection of the peritoneal fluid. The presence of bacteria on Gram stain of the initial fluid aspirate is not necessary for the diagnosis of peritonitis. Deterioration in mental status suggests impending hepatic coma. The treatment of bacterial peritonitis with gentamicin and clindamycin is preferable to the use of either agent alone. Intestinal aerobes that may be involved in peritonitis are sensitive to gentamicin; anaerobes, including most forms of *Bacteroides fragilis,* are sensitive to clindamycin.

60. The answer is A (1, 2, 3). *(Isselbacher, ed 9. p 200. Wilcocks, ed 17. pp 272-274.)* Trichuriasis is usually asymptomatic, although heavy infection may cause severe inflammation of the entire colon and rectum leading to dysentery and rectal prolapse. Epigastric and right lower quadrant pain with abdominal distension and flatulence may be found. Diagnosis of trichuriasis is made by finding characteristic eggs in the stool.

61. The answer is C (2, 4). *(Isselbacher, ed 9. p 607.)* The fatality rate in patients over the age of 12 with bacteremic pneumococcal pneumonia is 18 percent. The rate is significantly higher in patients who are over the age of 50, especially in patients with chronic disorders including cardiovascular disease, chronic bronchopulmonary and hepatic disease, diabetes, and renal insufficiency. The vaccine is recommended for all patients with sickle-cell disease who are more than two years old. Unfortunately, the vaccine is of little use in children under the age of two, who respond poorly to polysaccharide antigens, a circumstance that makes it difficult to protect them from many of the serious bacterial diseases that particularly affect this age group (e.g., *Hemophilus influenzae,* Group B *Streptococcus, Meningococcus*). Severe Arthus's reactions can develop if the antigen is administered more frequently than every three years. The vaccine is 80 to 90 percent efficient in adults. Patients without normal splenic function are susceptible to overwhelming pneumococcal septicemia with disseminated intravascular coagulation. In such patients, the vaccine is particularly useful.

62. The answer is E (all). *(Isselbacher, ed 9. pp 736-737. Youmans, pp 308-309, 376, 385.)* Infectious diseases of the central nervous system include cryptococcosis, coccidioidomycosis, nocardiosis, and mucormycosis. *Cryptococcus neoformans* characteristically causes a subacute or chronic meningitis, while *Coccidioides immitis* causes a more fulminant meningitis. *Nocardia asteroides* causes intracerebral abscesses. Presumably, these three microorganisms reach the central nervous system hematogenously from a primary pulmonary infection, which in the case of cryptococcosis may be inapparent. Fungi of the family Mucoraceae, on the other hand, reach the central nervous system via the sinuses and orbits (rhinocerebral mucormycosis).

63. The answer is C (2, 4). *(Isselbacher, ed 9. p 1333. Stamey, Trans Am Assoc Genitourin Surg 61:27-34, 1969.)* The diagnosis of chronic bacterial prostatitis cannot be based on positive urine cultures since the diagnosis depends on localization of the infection to the prostate gland. Localization must be based on quantitative bacterial cultures of (1) the first voided urine (urethral), (2) midstream urine (bladder), and (3) post-prostatic massage urine. The reliability of this method is greatest when the bladder urine is sterile. Chronic prostatitis may occur without the characteristic symptom of perineal pain. Urinary tract infection (i.e., cystitis), one of the most common complications of chronic prostatitis, may mask its presence. Intravenous pyelography serves no purpose in the diagnosis of chronic bacterial prostatitis.

64. The answer is E (all). *(Benenson, ed 12. pp 330-331. Isselbacher, ed 9. pp 894-895.)* There is no direct transmission of the larva of *Trichinella spiralis* to humans. Humans must eat the flesh of an animal in which there are encysted trichinae. The most important reservoir of such cysts is the hog, not cattle. The control of pork products is therefore of major importance in the prevention of human trichinosis.

65. The answer is A (1, 2, 3). *(Isselbacher, ed 9. pp 685-688.) Clostridium perfringens, C. tetani,* and *C. botulinum* all cause wound infections. *C. perfringens* may cause anaerobic cellulitis or myositis (gas gangrene). *C. tetani* and *C. botulinum* produce neurotoxins that have distinctive effects, but signs of local infection may be minimal. Tetanus toxin causes prolonged muscle spasms of flexor and extensor muscle groups. The masseter and respiratory muscles may be involved producing lockjaw and respiratory paralysis, respectively. *C. botulinum* toxin causes cranial nerve and symmetrical descending skeletal muscle paralysis; however, sensory function is not affected. Wound botulism is very rare; eight cases had been reported in the United States through January 1973. All clostridial wound infections require extensive debridement. For *C. tetani* and *C. botulinum* infections, antitoxin is given as well (preceded by skin testing for allergy since the antitoxin is produced in horses). Patients with any type of wound must be considered for tetanus prophylaxis. Adults are considered adequately immunized if they have completed a three-dose primary immunization series within ten years, or if they have received such a series earlier and been given a booster within ten years. Inadequately immunized patients should receive a booster if they completed the primary series, or a series of boosters if they did not. Hyperimmune antitetanus gamma globulin should be given only to patients who either have tetanus or have tetanus-prone wounds and have received either no previous immunization or only a single dose.

66. The answer is E (all). *(Isselbacher, ed 9. pp 738-739.) Histoplasma capsulatum* is an airborne microorganism causing primary infection of the lung. Lymphatic spread to regional lymph nodes and hematogenous spread to the liver and spleen are common. Infection in all these sites is suppressed by the immune response. A small number of affected patients may suffer relapse associated with hepatosplenomegaly and fever. This type of chronic disseminated histoplasmosis may be mistaken for a lymphoma. Disseminated infection may involve the adrenals, endocardium, pericardium, oropharynx, and larynx, as well as the meninges. Chronic pulmonary histoplasmosis resembles chronic pulmonary tuberculosis and may be associated with cavities.

67. The answer is E (all). *(Isselbacher, ed 9. pp 739-740.)* *Coccidioides immitis* has been found in certain semi-arid and arid regions of Arizona, Texas, and New Mexico, as well as in Mexico and some parts of Central and South America. Persons entering these regions from nonendemic areas are liable to become infected with this organism, which causes fever, malaise, dry cough, chest pain, night sweats, and anorexia. A macular or urticarial skin rash may be present within the first day or two of infection. Erythema nodosum or erythema multiforme and arthralgias may occur three days to three weeks after the onset of symptoms. The combination of erythema nodosum, arthralgias, and pneumonia represents the classic syndrome of valley fever (primary coccidioidomycosis). Headache and stiff neck occur much less commonly. Risk of dissemination from a pulmonary focus is very high in Filipinos and blacks.

68. The answer is C (2, 4). *(Isselbacher, ed 9. p 610. Waldvogel, N Engl J Med 282:198-206, 260-266, 316-322, 1970.)* Primary subacute osteomyelitis (Brodie's abscess) is a localized, indolent infection usually caused by *Staphylococcus aureus.* The lytic lesion, surrounded by an area of increased bone density (osteosclerosis), is seen almost always in the metaphyseal area of long bones; rarely, it may penetrate into the epiphysis or be found in the diaphysis. Bone cultures and characteristic histologic findings are necessary to confirm the diagnosis of primary subacute osteomyelitis and to eliminate malignancy as a cause of a lesion. Osteomyelitis of the frontal bone, associated with a history of disease in the frontal sinus, can present as a swelling over the frontal sinus preceded by cortical breakthrough and abscess formation under the periosteum (Pott's puffy tumor).

69. The answer is A (1, 2, 3). *(Isselbacher, ed 9. pp 721-727. Sparling, N Engl J Med 284:642-652, 1971.)* Biological false-positive reactions for syphilis have been reported in individuals who have systemic lupus erythematosus (SLE) and related connective tissue disorders, as well as conditions involving abnormal globulins. But false-positive reactions are considered to be rare in pregnancy. Patients who have SLE with or without a positive VDRL test also are reported to have atypical positive fluorescent treponemal antibody absorption (FTA-ABS) reactions; the only test that conclusively distinguishes a false-positive reaction from syphilis in this population remains the *Treponema pallidum* immobilization. Positivity here should be taken as evidence of disease. In a young person, a negative FTA-ABS rules out acquired syphilis; however, in older individuals who have late syphilis this test is occasionally negative.

70. The answer is C (2, 4). *(Isselbacher, ed 9. p 542. Yow, Medicine 52:305-309, 1973.)* The gram-negative enteric organisms, *Escherichia coli, Proteus,* and *Klebsiella pneumoniae*, comprise an important category of etiologic agents in neonatal meningitis. However, the group B *Streptococcus*, part of the normal flora of the human vagina, is now the major cause of meningitis in the first 30 days of life, a fact that is infrequently appreciated. Initial antibiotic selection should provide coverage for both gram-positive and gram-negative pathogens. A combination of ampicillin and an aminoglycoside constitutes effective initial therapy pending results of cultures.

71. The answer is D (4). *(Isselbacher, ed 9. pp 610-611. Knight, DM August: 27, 1976. Lerner, DM February: 22, 1975.)* A variety of bacteria may become secondary invaders after an episode of influenza, but for reasons not clear the association with *Staphylococcus aureus* and *Diplococcus pneumoniae* is greatest. Because mortality rates from secondary infection are high, the clinician should be on the alert for these organisms in cases of suspected influenza infection. Sensitivity to penicillin cannot be assumed for *S. aureus*.

72. The answer is E (all). *(Isselbacher, ed 9. pp 1965-1967. Karandanis, Arch Intern Med 135:1145-1149, 1975.)* In the case of an unruptured brain abscess, the spinal fluid culture is negative owing to the absence of an abscess-ventricular communication. Carotid arteriography, done early in the course of the disease, may be interpreted either as normal or as showing cerebritis or vasculitis. Repeat studies at a later time almost invariably demonstrate the mass lesion. Brain scan, however, is the most sensitive procedure in detecting early brain abscess and, of the methods listed in the question, would be the most likely to be abnormal if the presumptive diagnosis for the patient presented were correct.

73. The answer is D (4). *(Isselbacher, ed 9. pp 743, 1965.)* Patients who have cavernous sinus thrombosis with obstruction of the ophthalmic vein and involvement of cranial nerves III, IV, V, and VI are acutely ill and present characteristic eye findings of proptosis, chemosis, edema, and pain. Extension of the lesion through the intercavernous sinus to the contralateral sinus can be rapid. Although the commonest offending organism is *Staphylococcus aureus*, antibiotic therapy also should include coverage for *Proteus* and *Pseudomonas*. While mucormycosis and orbital cellulitis both enter the initial differential diagnosis of the patient discussed in the question, rapid spread of the lesion to the other eye in these disorders is uncommon.

74. The answer is D (4). *(Hunter, ed 5. pp 553-558. Isselbacher, ed 9. pp 907-911.)* In the patient presented in the question, a rectal biopsy to confirm the existence of *Schistosoma mansoni* eggs is not needed before treatment, because the diagnosis is already apparent. Niridazole is acceptable treatment for schistosomiasis and is widely used. The life cycle of *S. mansoni* involves an intermediate snail host; hence the eggs being excreted by this patient are not infectious for his siblings. Therefore, the patient is not a public health hazard unless he returns to a community where the cycle can perpetuate itself.

75. The answer is B (1, 3). *(Acton, pp 195-201. Isselbacher, ed 9. pp 801-804.)* Herpes zoster (shingles) usually is **unilateral** in distribution, causing a vesicular skin eruption that often halts abruptly at the midline of its dermatomal pattern. Despite a distinct association with Hodgkin's disease, zoster is not limited to this group of patients. Nevertheless, attempts to define an underlying lymphoproliferative disorder are indicated because of this association. Frequently, pain along affected dermatomes persists for many weeks after the skin lesion has disappeared.

76. The answer is B (1, 3). *(Isselbacher, ed 9. pp 1228-1229.)* Primary lung abscess can occur at any age and is associated with the loss of the gag reflex, leading to aspiration. In the younger population, epilepsy and drug abuse are leading causes of loss of gag reflex. The average number of organisms cultured from transtracheal or transthoracic lung puncture aspirates is three. The organisms, a mixture of anaerobes and aerobes, are streptococci, *Fusobacterium*, and *Bacteroides* species. The significance of anaerobic organisms in expectorated sputum cannot be assessed since they are part of the normal flora. "Reinfection" tuberculosis, which also characteristically presents as a cavity, usually affects an upper lobe rather than a dependent pulmonary segment. Drenching night sweats can occur with many severe systemic infections besides tuberculosis. Successful medical treatment of primary lung abscess now can be achieved with a combination of antibiotics, therapeutic bronchoscopy, and vigorous pulmonary toilet. Penicillin continues to be the antibiotic of choice. In the penicillin-sensitive patient, either clindamycin or chloramphenicol is effective. Bronchopleural fistula and empyema may occur in association with lung abscess, as they did in the patient presented in the question, whose x-rays can be observed to disclose an air-fluid level crossing the entire hemithorax. Drainage of the pleural space is mandatory in such cases.

77-81. The answers are: 77-E, 78-E, 79-A, 80-C, 81-C. *(Isselbacher, ed 9. p 579. Moellering, N Engl J Med 294:24-28, 1976.)* The cephalosporins are broad-spectrum antibacterials active against gram-positive and gram-negative species. They are resistant to penicillinase (beta-lactamase) and hence possess substantial antistaphylococcal activity. They also are effective against most streptococci other than enterococci. All cephalosporins are resistant in varying degrees to hydrolysis by a variety of beta-lactamases produced by staphylococci.

Cephalothin, the prototype of this class of antibiotics, remains one of the most effective cephalosporins against susceptible bacteria. It is highly resistant to beta lactamases.

Cephaloridine has lost favor because of its marked nephrotoxicity, yet it is the only cephalosporin approved for clinical use that achieves significant levels in the cerebrospinal fluid of patients who have inflamed meninges.

Cefazolin has the major advantages of being well tolerated after intramuscular administration and of achieving high blood levels. It has a long half-life and appears to be superior to other cephalosporins in reaching bile. Cefazolin is currently in widespread use although several reports of its failure to cure staphylococcal endocarditis have appeared.

Cephalexin is one of several orally-effective cephalosporins. Although this drug is expensive, it has a place in the management of urinary tract infection.

82-85. The answers are: 82-A, 83-A, 84-B, 85-A. *(Isselbacher, ed 9. p 572.)* Infections of renal parenchymal or perinephric areas are characterized by varied histories, symptoms, and clinical findings. Renal cortical abscesses almost invariably follow either an apparent or occult staphylococcal bacteremia, although pyuria is usually absent. The affected patient generally presents with fever, leukocytosis, and flank pain, but has no underlying renal disease.

In contrast, abscesses of the renal medulla are often associated with underlying kidney disease such as renal or ureteral calculi or pyelonephritis. Pyuria and gram-negative organisms on smear are typical of medullary abscesses.

Although perinephric abscess in the past usually followed a bacteremia from staphylococcal or streptococcal infections, today it is seen most commonly in association with ureteral calculi, hydronephrosis, noncalculus renal infections, and diabetes. It is notable that the organisms responsible for perinephric abscesses are predominantly those gram-negative enteric species associated with pyelonephritis. Thus, antibiotic therapy must provide for these organisms when the specific pathogen is not known. Perinephric abscess is diagnosed by demonstration of a mass on intravenous pyelography confirmed by renal arteriography. The urine in perinephric abscess may be unremarkable in the absence of an associated stone or pyelonephritis.

86-90. The answers are: 86-E, 87-C, 88-B, 89-D, 90-A. *(Isselbacher, ed 9. pp 736-739, 742. Youmans, pp 375-405.)* Infections caused by *Cryptococcus neoformans, Histoplasma capsulatum, Coccidioides immitus, Aspergillus fumigatus,* and *Blastomyces dermatitidis* in some cases are known, and in others believed, to be transmitted by inhalation of airborne microorganisms or spores. Lymphatic spread to regional lymph nodes and hematogenous dissemination to extra-pulmonary sites are common. The immune response in patients who have intact host defenses quickly suppresses or eradicates infection. But in patients who have lymphoma or are receiving corticosteroids, the pulmonary or extra-pulmonary infection may be progressive.

C. neoformans has been isolated from pigeon droppings around the world. *C. immitis* is found in arid and semi-arid regions of southwestern United States and may be carried great distances by fomites.

H. capsulatum exists primarily in the Mississippi and Ohio River Valleys as well as in areas of West Virginia, Virginia, Pennsylvania, and Maryland; it is isolated from soil high in organic content, especially bird droppings. The spores may be stirred up by excavations or demolition.

A. fumigatus has been isolated from decaying vegetation around the world. Invasive infection occurs almost exclusively in compromised hosts. Saprophytic endobronchial infection may occur in patients who have bronchiectasis or pulmonary cavities. Hypersensitivity to *Aspergillus* may lead to episodes of wheezing and obstructive lung disease (bronchopulmonary aspergillosis).

The epidemiology and pathophysiology of *B. dermatitidis* infections are not fully understood. Cutaneous manifestations predominate but pulmonary, disseminated, and genital tract infection may occur as well.

91-95. The answers are: 91-C, 92-D, 93-A, 94-E, 95-B. *(Isselbacher, ed 9. pp 581-582. Kucers, ed 3. pp 172, 264, 283-290, 304.)* Side effects from antibiotics can be serious. Liver damage caused by erythromycin and isoniazid is well recognized. However, liver damage has also been associated with rifampin therapy. A combination of rifampin and isoniazid—now widely recommended as the treatment of choice for active tuberculosis—not surprisingly is associated with increased hepatotoxicity.

All tetracyclines may provoke photosensitivity reactions, but the long-acting tetracyclines are more likely to produce this side effect. The long-acting variety has a markedly prolonged plasma half-life because of a propensity for protein-binding (greater than 90 percent) as compared to other tetracyclines and tetracycline itself (70 percent). Demeclocycline, one of the long-acting tetracyclines, is widely recommended for the prophylactic avoidance of traveler's diarrhea. Thus, it is not surprising that a number of cases of photosensitivity have developed in vacationers.

Ototoxicity and vestibular disturbances are among the most serious of antibiotic side effects. Vancomycin can produce irreversible deafness, especially in oliguric patients. This drug is widely used because of its suitability in patients who are allergic to penicillin. Owing to the necessity for intravenous administration of vancomycin, thrombophlebitis is a common side effect of this agent. Transient chills, fever, and renal toxicity are also associated with vancomycin. Nephrotoxicity can best be avoided by carefully relating the dose of the drug to renal function. For example, it may be satisfactory to give some patients with renal disease a single dose of 1 g of vancomycin every week to ten days.

Chloramphenicol, a bacteriostatic agent, would perhaps be the most useful antibiotic available were it not for its side effects. Its direct side effects include development of aplastic anemia (1 in 25,000 cases) and inhibition of protein synthesis associated with doses that exceed 2 g a day. While this effect is severe, it is reversible. Clinically, this complication is recognized by the development of leukopenia, anemia, and thrombocytopenia in association with high serum iron levels and saturation of serum transferrin. Chloramphenicol also is antagonistic to drugs, such as penicillin, that reduce bacteria populations by impairing bacterial cell division.

96-99. The answers are: 96-C, 97-E, 98-A, 99-D. *(Isselbacher, ed 9. pp 658, 685, 691, 711.)* Brucellosis (undulant fever) is primarily due to infection with *Brucella melitensis, B. suis,* and *B. abortus*. The animal reservoirs of these organisms are goats, hogs, and cattle, respectively. The disease is rarely transmitted from person to person. On a worldwide basis, *B. melitensis* is the most common cause of brucellosis, secondary to the ingestion of goat's milk cheese. Affected patients may suffer from chronic ill health manifested by (1) weakness and fatigue; (2) mental depression; (3) psychoneuroses; and (4) both mental depression and psychoneuroses. They have vague aches and pains but no actual physical findings.

Mycobacterium leprae (Hansen's bacillus) multiplies only in the cooler areas of the body. One of the favored sites is the nasal mucosa; chronic sinusitis frequently follows. Other commonly affected areas include the skin and the peripheral nerves; disseminated leprosy, involving internal organs, does not occur. The armadillo, common in the Southwest part of the United States, also suffers from leprosy associated with the human *M. leprae* organism. However, because of the animal's extremely low body temperature, disseminated infection does occur. Armadillos are proving a useful model in which to study the immune response to the organism.

Herpes labialis, which can follow a number of bacterial infections, occurs in as many as 20 percent of patients with meningococcal infections. Recurrent, and frequently localized, infections associated with intermittent shedding of virus occur in many patients. The virus is able to replicate in many tissues and cells and, once having assumed an intracellular location, is immune to antiherpes antibodies. Why gram-positive organisms, such as pneumococci and meningococci, can activate clinical infections is unknown. Although stress and menstruation frequently are noted in association with exacerbation of herpes labialis infection, the responsible mechanisms remain unclear.

The pathologic changes produced by *Clostridium* result from the ability of these organisms to form an exotoxin that kills tissue cells. At least a dozen distinct extracellular toxins are elaborated by *C. perfringens*, of which alpha toxin (lecithinase) is the most important—it can produce a hemolytic anemia with incredible rapidity. *C. perfringens* is responsible for most clostridial infections of the uterus and when ingested with contaminated food, commonly causes a severe enterocolitis. *C. perfringens* is a nonmotile encapsulated organism. Boiling will almost always destroy the spores of this organism.

100-104. The answers are: 100-C, 101-D, 102-A, 103-B, 104-E. *(Isselbacher, ed 9. pp 556, 703-704, 1213, 1538. Youmans, pp 271-291.)* Acute tuberculous pneumonia (figure C appearing in the question) may occur when a large apical tuberculous cavity ruptures, spilling large numbers of organisms into the lower airways. The isolation of *Staphylococcus aureus* from the sputum is not, by itself, conclusive evidence of staphylococcal pneumonia. In most cases of tuberculous pneumonia, cultures and smears for *Mycobacterium tuberculosis* are positive.

Viral pneumonia (figure D) characteristically causes a diffuse pulmonary infiltrate. The coexistence of a vesicular skin rash may suggest the etiology. Varicella infection or herpes occurs with distressing frequency in victims of Hodgkin's disease and other lymphomas.

Aspergillus fumigatus may cause saprophytic endobronchial infection (mycetoma) in patients who have residual pulmonary cavities (figures A_1 and A_2). Characteristically, affected patients will have recurrent episodes of hemoptysis. The silhouette of the mycetoma (or fungus ball) may be seen in the cavity. Laminograms may be required to identify this type of infection.

Allergy to *A. fumigatus* may cause recurrent episodes of bronchospasm and eventually chronic obstructive lung disease (bronchopulmonary aspergillosis—figures B_1 and B_2).

Owing to its association with such diseases as systemic lupus erythematosus and polyarteritis nodosa (or to its treatment with high dose corticosteroids), thrombotic thrombocytopenic purpura is conjectured to arise from a compromised host defense system. In patients afflicted with the disorders mentioned, opportunistic infections are likely. *Nocardia asteroides* may cause a necrotizing pulmonary infection with abscess formation (figure E_1). Signs or symptoms of an associated cerebral abscess may suggest the diagnosis. Although sputum cultures often are positive, a lung biopsy may be required to confirm the diagnosis (figure E_2).

105-109. The answers are: 105-A, 106-A, 107-D, 108-C, 109-E. *(Hansten, ed 4. pp 40, 57, 130, 187. Isselbacher, ed 9. pp 379-381, 1557.)* The trend to the utilization of combination drugs makes it imperative that clinicians be conscious of possible interactions among them. One important interaction is the effect of some antibiotics on anticoagulants. For instance, broad-spectrum antibiotics, such as tetracycline, enhance the anticoagulant effect of dicumarol by decreasing the number of vitamin K-producing bacteria in the gut. Vitamin K is essential for the production by the liver of clotting factor II (prothrombin). Chloramphenicol causes an increase in the anticoagulant effect of dicumarol by interfering with the hepatic metabolism of the drug. In addition to the increased risk of bleeding during the course of an infection in a patient who is receiving both anticoagulant and antibiotic therapy, cessation of the antibiotic may be associated with an increased risk of clotting as the level of circulating anticoagulants is reduced. Many commonly used drugs, however, have the opposite effect of **reducing** the efficiency of oral anticoagulants. Such drugs include the barbiturates, digitoxin, quinidine, dexamethasone, and metyrapone.

Patients receiving the antibacterial agent, trimethoprim, in combination with the thiazide diuretics or furosemide may experience an increased incidence of thrombocytopenia. It is known that thiazide diuretics can act as myelosuppressive drugs, as can ethanol and estrogens. The sulfonamides, including trimethoprim, are suspected but not proven to produce immunologically mediated destruction of platelets.

The ability of allopurinol to effect partial inhibition of xanthine oxidase also makes this drug useful for the treatment of gout. It often is administered in situations, such as malignancies, in which rapid turnover of cells is associated with the release of large amounts of uric acid, thus incurring the risk of gouty symptoms. Allopurinol administered in combination with azathioprine (a 6-mercaptopurine derivative) can result in a life-threatening toxicity that produces bone marrow suppression. Azathioprine is normally converted to 6-mercaptopurine, an active metabolite, which is partially inactivated by the enzyme xanthine oxidase.

110-112. The answers are: 110-C, 111-B, 112-A. *(Hansten, ed 4. pp 75, 148, 167. Isselbacher, ed 9. pp 379-380.)* Combinations of drugs may have unexpected effects. The gastrointestinal absorption of one of two combined drugs may be reduced, as occurs when digitails and tetracycline are combined with neomycin and antacids, respectively.

Increased toxic effects from one or both drugs also may result from combined drug therapy, as in the following examples: rifampin with isoniazid (increased hepatotoxicity); aminoglycosides with skeletal muscle relaxants (respiratory paralysis) and, possibly, also with ethacrynic acid or furosemide (increased nephrotoxicity); rifampin with halothane (increased hepatotoxicity);

and methoxyflurane with aminoglycosides or tetracycline (increased renal toxicity).

Finally, the half-life of one of the two drugs may be prolonged if they share a common metabolic pathway. In this manner, chloramphenicol prolongs the half-life of barbiturates, phenytoin (Dilantin), warfarin (Coumadin), and tolbutamide; isoniazid prolongs the half-life of phenytoin, and sulfonamides prolong the half-life of tolbutamide.

113-117. The answers are: 113-A, 114-C, 115-D, 116-B, 117-E. *(Isselbacher, ed 9. pp 609, 648, 665, 677, 692.)* The most common causes of food-borne illness in the United States are *Clostridia perfringens* and *Staphylococcus aureus*. Both bacteria produce toxins in food during preparation. The clostridial food toxin is heat-labile, while the staphylococcal toxin is heat-stable. Fever is uncommon in illnesses caused by these toxins, which also is true of other toxin-mediated types of illness carried by food. Lower intestinal symptoms predominate with illness from *Clostridia*-contaminated food, whereas upper intestinal symptoms predominate with illness from staphylococcal-contaminated food.

Ingestion of bacteria with subsequent invasion of the intestinal mucosa has been associated with *Shigella sonnei* and other *Shigella* species, *Salmonella typhi*, *Vibrio parahaemolyticus*, and *Yersinia enterocolitica*. Illness caused by these microorganisms in food is generally associated with fever, abdominal pain, and diarrhea.

Severe cramps and bloody diarrhea are associated with the *Shigella* infections. *Vibrio parahaemolyticus* has been associated with contaminated crabs caught in the Chesapeake Bay, and high salt concentrations in culture media are required to isolate this microorganism. *Yersinia enterocolitica*, which commonly causes infection in northern Europe, has recently been identified in the United States. Symptoms of infection with this organism may mimic appendicitis.

Rheumatology

DIRECTIONS: Each question below contains five suggested answers. Choose the **one best** response to each question.

118. A 65-year-old woman who has a 12-year history of symmetrical polyarthritis is admitted to the hospital. Physical examination reveals splenomegaly, ulcerations over the anterior shins, and synovitis of the wrists, shoulders, and knees. Laboratory values demonstrate a white blood cell count of $2500/mm^3$ and a rheumatoid factor titer of 1:4096. This patient's white blood cell differential count is likely to reveal

(A) pancytopenia
(B) lymphopenia
(C) granulocytopenia
(D) lymphocytosis
(E) basophilia

119. Hereditary deficiency of C2 may be associated with

(A) an increased incidence of bacterial infections
(B) arthritis, photosensitivity, and glomerulonephritis
(C) impaired granulocyte function
(D) agammaglobulinemia
(E) chronic granulomatous hepatitis

120. A 35-year-old man complains of progressive low back pain. He has also developed moderate deafness over the last five years and has had numerous attacks of prostatitis. Physical examination reveals moderate kyphosis and a bluish discoloration of the cartilage of his ears. The metabolic abnormality associated with this patient's disease can be identified by demonstrating

(A) calcium pyrophosphate in synovial fluid
(B) basophilic stippling of red blood cells
(C) homogentisic acid in urine
(D) tryptophan in urine
(E) delta-aminolevulenic acid in urine

121. Reiter's syndrome is characterized by all the following features EXCEPT

(A) cardiac conduction abnormalities
(B) iritis
(C) spondylitis
(D) aseptic meningitis
(E) hematuria

122. True LE cells are best described as

(A) polymorphonuclear leukocytes that have ingested nuclei from other cells
(B) polymorphonuclear leukocytes that have ingested lymphocytes
(C) monocytes that have ingested nuclei from other cells
(D) monocytes that have formed rosettes with erythrocytes
(E) hematoxylin bodies

123. Arthritis of the temporomandibular joint may be caused by all the following diseases EXCEPT

(A) gout
(B) ankylosing spondylitis
(C) adult rheumatoid arthritis
(D) juvenile rheumatoid arthritis
(E) osteoarthritis

124. A 25-year-old debilitated man who admits to frequent self administration of intravenous drugs presents at an emergency room with a flat, nonspecific erythematous rash on his arms and trunk. He gives a one-week history of pain and swelling in the fingers of both hands and a two-day history of urticaria. He has a chronic cough but his chief complaint is of pain and swelling, of 24 hours duration, in his right knee. The pain is moderately severe with movement. The patient has a temperature of 37.8°C (100°F) and limitation of flexion at the metacarpophalangeal and proximal interphalangeal joints of both hands. A small effusion is noted in the right knee. The most likely diagnosis of this man's disorder would be

(A) gonococcal arthritis
(B) rheumatoid arthritis
(C) rheumatoid arthritis complicated by a septic arthritis
(D) tuberculous arthritis
(E) viral hepatitis complicated by arthritis

125. Chondrocalcinosis is best identified by which of the following clinical procedures?

(A) Routine x-rays of joints
(B) Arthrography
(C) Synovial fluid aspiration
(D) Arthroscopy
(E) Bone biopsy

126. Which of the following statements about anserine bursitis is true?

(A) It causes pain on climbing stairs
(B) It causes "locked knee"
(C) It is associated with hyperthyroidism
(D) It is usually limited to childhood
(E) It is a complication of intra-articular steroid therapy

127. A 25-year-old man awakens with excruciating pain in the first metatarsophalangeal joint of his right foot. His physician identifies needle-shaped, negatively birefringent crystals in synovial fluid aspirated from the affected joint. The most desirable therapy for this patient would be

(A) allopurinol, 300 mg, and colchicine, 1.6 mg daily
(B) colchicine, 3 mg twice a day
(C) sulfinpyrazone, 400 mg daily
(D) indomethacin, 200-250 mg daily in divided doses
(E) salicylate, 3800 mg daily in divided doses

DIRECTIONS: Each question below contains four suggested answers of which **one** or **more** is correct. Choose the answer:

A	if	**1, 2, and 3**	are correct
B	if	**1 and 3**	are correct
C	if	**2 and 4**	are correct
D	if	**4**	is correct
E	if	**1, 2, 3, and 4**	are correct

128. A 17-year-old white male high school student seeks medical advice because of recurrent low back pain and stiffness that last for a few days after each football game and extended practice session. The youth is otherwise healthy, has no family history of joint problems, and no abnormal physical findings. Radiographic examination of his spine and sacroiliac joints reveals no abnormalities. Serology studies are not helpful and the patient's erythrocyte sedimentation rate is 13 mm/hr (Westergren). However, the patient is found to have the histocompatibility antigen HLA-B27 on his leukocytes. With this information, the physician can now advise his patient that

(1) it would be advisable to have an x-ray examination of his large bowel
(2) he should have an annual slit-lamp examination of his eye
(3) he should have phenylbutazone daily for the next year while his physician observes him closely for signs of developing spondylitis
(4) he has a 25 percent chance of developing significant spondylitis

129. Giant cell arteritis is recognized to be a cause of

(1) diffuse proliferative glomerulonephritis
(2) aortic aneurysms
(3) complement activation
(4) blindness

130. Paget's disease of bone includes which of the following complications?

(1) Deafness
(2) High-output heart failure
(3) Sarcoma
(4) Development of arteriovenous fistulas

131. Tietze's syndrome is characterized by which of the following statements?

(1) It usually involves only a single costochondral cartilage
(2) It usually follows an injury to the chest wall
(3) It is accompanied by swelling
(4) It may accompany epidemic pleurodynia caused by group B coxsackievirus infection

132. Elevated blood levels of creatine phosphokinase may be found in association with

(1) myocardial infarction
(2) hypothyroidism
(3) polymyositis
(4) polymyalgia rheumatica

133. Adult rheumatoid arthritis is characterized by radiologic findings that include

(1) juxta-articular erosions
(2) periarticular osteopenia
(3) loss of joint space
(4) periostitis

134. Correct statements about the etiology and pathogenesis of degenerative joint disease include which of the following?

(1) Osteoarthritic cartilage undergoes increased metabolic activity and increased cell division, indicating that increased degradation and increased synthesis of cartilage matrix occur concurrently
(2) Degenerative disease of the wrists, elbows, and shoulders is relatively uncommon unless these joints are subjected to occupational trauma
(3) Extensive degenerative joint disease is found late in the course of acromegaly
(4) The usual laboratory tests show no abnormalities in degenerative joint disease

135. Relapsing polychondritis, a disease of unknown cause that leads to inflammation and destruction of cartilage, is characterized by which of the following clinical findings?

(1) The ears or nose may become swollen and tender
(2) Hearing loss may occur
(3) Hoarseness and recurrent pulmonary infections are common
(4) The disease is unresponsive to anti-inflammatory therapy

136. Sjögren's syndrome may occur in association with which of the following diseases?

(1) Scleroderma
(2) Polymyositis
(3) Systemic lupus erythematosus
(4) Rheumatoid arthritis

137. Extra-articular manifestations of rheumatoid arthritis include

(1) Bouchard's nodes
(2) subcutaneous nodules
(3) glomerulonephritis
(4) pleural effusions

138. Rheumatoid factor is generally an antibody of the IgM class that will react with

(1) latex particles
(2) aggregated rabbit gammaglobulin
(3) bentonite particles
(4) aggregated human gammaglobulin

SUMMARY OF DIRECTIONS

A	B	C	D	E
1, 2, 3 only	1. 3 only	2, 4 only	4 only	All are correct

139. Clinical manifestations of Behçet's disease include

(1) aphthous stomatitis
(2) genital ulceration
(3) iritis
(4) thrombophlebitis

140. Correct statements about osteoarthritis include which of the following?

(1) It has an approximately equal incidence in men and women
(2) It is usually associated with osteoporosis
(3) It may be initiated by acute trauma to a joint
(4) It is usually associated with synovial fluid white blood cell counts greater than $10{,}000/mm^3$

141. Morton's metatarsalgia is associated with which of the following conditions?

(1) Plantar warts
(2) Footdrop
(3) Diabetes mellitus
(4) Compression of the superficial branch of the plantar nerve

142. A 50-year-old coal miner develops pain in both knees. Which of the following pieces of information will help to determine whether he has osteoarthritis or rheumatoid arthritis?

(1) Knowledge of his occupation
(2) The presence or absence of morning stiffness
(3) The erythrocyte sedimentation rate
(4) Synovial fluid viscosity

143. A 32-year-old woman afflicted with paroxysmal atrial tachycardia had been treated with procainamide for two years when she began to complain of fever, pleuritic chest pain, arthralgias, and fatigue. These symptoms persisted for two months. Which of the following tests would be useful in determining the etiology of this syndrome?

(1) Determination of the titer of antibodies to procainamide
(2) Determination of antinative DNA antibodies
(3) Determination of C3 level
(4) Fluorescent antinuclear antibody test

DIRECTIONS: The group of questions below consists of lettered choices followed by several numbered items. For each numbered item select the **one** lettered choice with which it is **most** closely associated. Each lettered choice may be used once, more than once, or not at all.

Questions 144-148

For each set of synovial fluid data that follows, select the disease with which it is most likely to be associated.

(A) Degenerative joint disease
(B) Pseudogout
(C) Systemic lupus erythematosus
(D) Reiter's syndrome
(E) Rheumatoid arthritis

	Mucin Clot	Fibrin Clot	Appearance	Total WBC (per mm^3)	Percent Polys	Synovial Fluid Complement	Glucose, % of Blood Level
144.	Poor	Large	Turbid	35,000	80	Normal	90
145.	Good	Small	Slightly Turbid	1,100	15	Normal	98
146.	Poor	Large	Turbid	50,000	70	Decreased	75
147.	Good	Large	Straw Colored	10,000	25	Decreased	75
148.	Fair	Large	Turbid	50,000	55	Increased	75

Rheumatology

Answers

118. The answer is C. *(Beeson, ed 15. p 193. Isselbacher, ed 9. p 1875.)* Felty's syndrome consists of a triad of rheumatoid arthritis, splenomegaly, and leukopenia. In contrast with the lymphopenia observed in patients who have systemic lupus erythematosus, the leukopenia of Felty's syndrome is related to a reduction in the number of circulating polymorphonuclear leukocytes. The mechanism of the granulocytopenia is poorly understood. Felty's syndrome tends to occur in individuals who have had active rheumatoid arthritis for a prolonged period. These patients commonly have other systemic features of rheumatoid disease such as nodules, skin ulcerations, the sicca complex, peripheral sensory and motor neuropathy, and arteritic lesions.

119. The answer is B. *(Isselbacher, ed 9. pp 322-324. Kohler, Ann Intern Med 82:420, 1975.)* Isolated deficiencies have been described for all proteins of the complement system with the exception of C8 and C9. Patients who have a C2 deficiency do not appear to have an increased susceptibility to infection. However, in patients genetically lacking this component, a syndrome closely resembling systemic lupus erythematosus has been described. These patients differ from patients who have the usual form of systemic lupus erythematosus in being more predisposed to photosensitivity. In addition, individuals lacking C2 tend to have absent or low titers of antinuclear antibodies and do not form deposits of C3 at the dermal-epidermal junction.

120. The answer is C. *(Isselbacher, ed 9. pp 468-469. McCarty, ed 9. pp 1262-1267.)* Spondylosis with back pain and kyphosis, chronic prostatitis, and deafness are all characteristic of ochronosis, a disease that results from a deficiency of homogentisic acid oxidase. In the absence of this enzyme, homogentisic acid appears in the urine. Urine that contains homogentisic acid gradually turns brownish-black on exposure to air as oxidation occurs. This color change can be accelerated by adding a few drops of sodium hydroxide to alkalinize the urine.

121. The answer is D. *(Isselbacher, ed 9. pp 1883-1884. McCarty, ed 9. pp 633-641.)* Reiter's syndrome, consisting of urethritis, arthritis, and conjunctivitis, may be accompanied by other characteristic manifestations including sacroiliitis, spondylitis, circinate balanitis, iritis, keratoderma blennorrhagicum, and shallow, painless, oral ulcerations. Reiter's syndrome frequently starts with a urethritis obtained from sexual exposure. The onset of symptoms such as arthritis, conjunctivitis, and mucocutaneous lesions occurs anywhere from a few days to four weeks after the development of urethritis. Cardiac conduction abnormalities, pericarditis, and peripheral neuropathy are less common features. Although most patients recover from the initial attack of Reiter's syndrome within several months, some develop a chronic illness that evolves into a picture indistinguishable from psoriatic arthritis or ankylosing spondylitis.

122. The answer is A. *(Isselbacher, ed 9. p 358. McCarty, ed 9. p 716.)* LE cells are produced when complement-fixing antinucleoprotein antibodies react with nuclei of injured cells. In the presence of complement, the nucleus from the injured cell is then phagocytosed by a polymorphonuclear leukocyte. The tart cell, a cell closely related to the LE cell, results from a similar mechanism, but in its case the phagocytosing cell is a monocyte. Tart cells are less specific for systemic lupus erythematosus than are true LE cells. True LE cells are found in approximately 50 percent of patients who have systemic lupus erythematosus, 5 percent of patients who have rheumatoid arthritis, and rarely if at all in normal individuals.

123. The answer is A. *(Isselbacher, ed 9. p 192. McCarty, ed 9. pp 989-990.)* Temporomandibular joint involvement is a classic feature of juvenile rheumatoid arthritis and, when present prior to closure of the epiphysis of the mandible, results in micrognathia. Adult rheumatoid arthritis frequently causes temporomandibular joint symptoms, and osteoarthritis and ankylosing spondylitis affect the joint in a smaller percentage of cases. Gout does not affect this particular joint.

124. The answer is E. *(Isselbacher, ed 9. p 1893.)* Arthritis is a relatively common manifestation of type B hepatitis, as is the occurrence of urticaria in the prodromal phase. Clinically detectable jaundice may not develop for a few days or even weeks after the onset of a severe arthritis, which tends to be migratory and involves both small and large joints. As the involvement in the hands is frequently symmetrical, it is easily confused with rheumatoid arthritis. The arthritis may be accompanied by a rash. Suspicion of a hepatitis-induced arthritis will be confirmed by the detection of abnormal liver functions, especially elevated liver enzymes, while Australia antigen—and perhaps antibody—will be detected in the serum and joint fluid in which complement levels may also be low, indicating active antigen-antibody complex deposition. Permanent joint damage may develop rapidly as a complication of septic arthritis. Early diagnosis with appropriate management of the arthritis is essential if this complication is to be avoided. Infectious arthritis can arise from viral, bacterial, and mycotic infections and although the diagnosis relies heavily on examination and culture of the joint fluid, these observations may not be immediately helpful. The following considerations are useful in making a differential diagnosis. *Hemophilus influenzae*, which frequently causes meningitis in children, is most often responsbile for a septic arthritis in this age group. Septic arthritis due to *Staphylococcus aureus* is now frequently encountered in drug-addicted persons who administer their drugs by an intravenous route. Gonococcal arthritis remains a disease of sexually active persons, usually women, who are particularly prone to develop a bacteremia at the time of menstruation. Bilateral and symmetrical synovial thickening of the joints of the hands and wrists is unusual in gonococcal arthritis, although skin rashes are common. Rheumatoid arthritis is more common in women than men but usually is not associated with a rash, although Still's disease occurring in adults features a generalized rash. Patients with rheumatoid arthritis who present with sudden localized pain and swelling should be carefully evaluated for a septic joint; underlying joint disease increases susceptibility to secondary septic involvement of a joint space. Bacterial sepsis usually presents with severe splinting and restriction of movement. Tuberculous arthritis, although now very rare, is more likely to arise in children than adults. Arthritis and inflammation around the infected joints develop slowly, with spine, hips, and knees being particularly susceptible. Symmetrical disease of the hands is rare in tuberculosis, while the thickened synovium found in this condition has a characteristic boggy or doughy feeling.

125. The answer is C. *(Committee of the American Rheumatism Association Section of The Arthritis Foundation, JAMA 224:104, 1973. Isselbacher, ed 9. p 1888.)* Chondrocalcinosis refers to the deposition of calcium-containing salts like calcium hydroxyapatite, calcium pyrophosphate, and calcium orthophosphate in articulating cartilage, detected radiologically as a thin line of calcification within the joint space. This condition may be asymptomatic or may be associated with attacks of inflammatory arthritis referred to as pseudogout, clinically indistinguishable from attacks of gouty arthritis related to crystals of sodium urate. The diagnosis of pseudogout is most readily made by identifying the crystals of calcium pyrophosphate in synovial fluid aspirated from affected joints.

126. The answer is A. *(Isselbacher, ed 9. p 1902. McCarty, ed 9. pp 996-997.)* Anserine bursitis is caused by inflammation of the sartorius bursa on the medial aspect of the tibia. It tends to occur in obese women and in association with osteoarthritis of the knee. Characteristically, pain from anserine bursitis is provoked by climbing stairs or by pressure at the site of the sartorius muscle. Relief may be obtained by the local injection of steroids.

127. The answer is D. *(Isselbacher, ed 9. pp 479-486.)* Appropriate therapy of acute gouty arthritis can be divided into two phases. In the first phase, the acute gouty inflammation is controlled by anti-inflammatory agents administered, usually, in conjunction with an analgesic agent in severe cases. In the second phase, the serum urate level is lowered by uricosuric agents or drugs designed to inhibit the development of uric acid. Traditionally, acute gouty inflammation has been controlled by giving colchicine on an hourly basis until a therapeutic response occurs. However, as many as 80 percent of gout patients cannot achieve satisfactory therapeutic levels with colchicine because of the toxicity of the drug. Recently, anti-inflammatory drugs such as indomethacin or phenylbutazone have been found to be equally as effective as colchicine and to have fewer of the gastrointestinal side effects frequently associated with colchicine. Allopurinol, a xanthine oxidase inhibitor, and the uricosuric agents, probenecid and sulfinpyrazone effectively reverse hyperuricemia, but do not relieve inflammation associated with acute attacks of gouty arthritis. The intense pain of gout may well require an initial dose of a narcotic analgesic to make the patient more comfortable while the anti-inflammatory agents have time to suppress the arthritis.

128. The answer is D (4). *(Isselbacher, ed 9. pp 1880-1882.)* The histocompatibility antigen HLA-B27 is the histocompatibility protein complex that represents the expression of the HLA-B27 allele situated at the B locus on the short arm of chromosome 6. This location is very close to the D locus of chromosome 6 which, apart from being responsible for the expression of D locus antigens on the surface of many cells, especially B cells and macrophages, is thought to be intimately associated with the various alleles that determine the appropriateness and efficiency of immunoregulatory function at the level of the T cell. When alleles of different loci are associated in the population more frequently than would be expected by chance, the phenomenon is termed linkage disequilibrium. HLA-B27 antigens are associated with ankylosing spondylitis because the HLA-B27 allele is associated by linkage disequilibrium with alleles near the D locus that failed to prevent the development of an inflammatory reaction in certain tissues such as the uveal tract of the eye, the vertebral column, joint spaces, and the urethral tract. The inflammation in these tissues is most commonly ascribed to defects in immunoregulation. Although 90 percent of patients with ankylosing spondylitis have the HLA-B27 gene, as opposed to seven percent of the normal white population, the presence of the gene in the absence of a family history and convincing manifestations of this disorder indicates a risk no greater than 25 percent for developing spondylitis. Only 20 to 30 percent of patients with definite spondylitis develop uveitis. Thus, routine examination of the eye in asymptomatic patients is not warranted. The HLA-B27 gene is found in 60 to 75 percent of patients with enteropathic spondylitis. However, the presence of the gene product *per se* is insufficient reason to examine the large bowel. The most likely diagnosis in the patient presented in the question is local traumatic injury associated with his athletic endeavors. Phenylbutazone, which can be effective in spondylitis, has side effects and is not recommended in the absence of a conclusive diagnosis.

129. The answer is C (2, 4). *(Isselbacher, ed 9. pp 354-355. Klein, Ann Intern Med 83:806-812, 1975.)* Giant cell arteritis is a form of necrotizing arteritis that occurs almost exclusively in elderly individuals. Lesions tend to be concentrated in one or more branches of a carotid artery, but may involve other vessels such as the aorta and the subclavian, renal, and mesenteric arteries. Involvement of the aorta can lead to formation of an aortic aneurysm that may rupture. Patients who have giant cell arteritis usually benefit from corticosteroid therapy. Immune complexes and low levels of complement are rarely found in association with giant cell arteritis, which does not have an established immunologic basis. Giant cell arteritis is a disease of the elderly. Frequently a prodrome, known as polymyalgia rheumatica, is diagnosable. Stiffness in the upper part of the neck and shoulders, and occasionally the upper arms, is characteristic of this syndrome. A biopsy of both temporal arteries in patients with asymptomatic temporal arteritis frequently will be positive in the presence of polymyalgia rheumatica. The characteristic onset of clinical arteritis—weight loss, malaise, fever, and anorexia—can ensue. Headache is a frequent symptom. This form of arteritis, which can lead to blindness, usually responds to corticosteroid therapy.

130. The answer is A (1, 2, 3). *(Isselbacher, ed 9. p 1860.)* Paget's disease is a condition in which focal areas of the skeleton develop an increased rate of bone turnover. At sites of involvement, rapid resorption of bone is accompanied by a compensating increase in new bone formation; either of the two processes may predominate, resulting in osteoporotic changes in the first case and sclerotic changes in the second. The skull may become enlarged and deafness may occur either from compression of the 8th cranial nerve as it passes through the auditory foramen or from direct pagetic involvement of the ossicles. High-output cardiac failure sometimes occurs in patients with Paget's disease. This is thought to be related to an increased rate of blood flow in the skin overlying involved bone. The most lethal complication in Paget's disease is sarcoma, which develops in less than 1 percent of affected patients. Arteriovenous fistulas have not been demonstrated.

131. The answer is B (1, 3). *(Isselbacher, ed 9. p 1902. McCarty, ed 9. pp 991-992.)* Tietze's syndrome is thought to be a form of costochondritis. Affected patients are characteristically found to have a painful swelling of a single upper costochondral junction. In a minority of cases, more than one level may be involved. The condition may run its course in a few days or become chronic and last for many months. The etiology is unknown; biopsy usually reveals normal cartilage, sometimes with inflammation in the surrounding soft tissue.

132. The answer is A (1, 2, 3). *(Beeson, ed 15. p 1232. Isselbacher, ed 9. p 1126.)* Creatine phosphokinase (CPK) is an enzyme found in high concentration in heart, skeletal muscle, and brain. Injury to muscle such as occurs in polymyositis or myocardial infarction releases this enzyme from the muscle cells, producing elevated levels in the circulation. CPK levels are also elevated in patients afflicted with hypothyroidism. Clinically, polymyalgia rheumatica is often confused with polymyositis because affected patients in both cases appear weak. However, careful strength testing of polymyalgia rheumatica patients reveals normal muscle power. CPK blood levels also help to distinguish between these two diseases since the level of the enzyme is normal in polymyalgia rheumatica but usually elevated in polymyositis.

133. The answer is A (1, 2, 3). *(Committee of the American Rheumatism Association Section of The Arthritis Foundation, JAMA 224:129, 1973. Isselbacher, ed 9. p 1876.)* The earliest radiologic abnormality usually observed in adult rheumatoid arthritis is periarticular osteopenia. This may be observed after inflammation has been present for only a few weeks. After a period of three to six months, extra-articular erosions and joint space narrowing may appear. Following a prolonged period, bony ankylosis may develop. Periostitis, common in juvenile rheumatoid arthritis and psoriatic arthritis, is uncommon in the adult form of rheumatoid arthritis.

134. The answer is E (all). *(Isselbacher, ed 9. pp 1894-1896.)* The major characteristics of degenerative joint disease are loss of joint cartilage and hypertrophy of bone. Within osteoarthritic cartilage, there is a marked increase in metabolic activity owing to the increased rate of destruction of cartilage accompanied by an increased synthesis of cartilage matrix. The increased proteolytic activity in the joint space is associated with higher than normal levels of proteases, particularly cathepsin D and similar hydrolases. As the disease progresses, cartilage is steadily lost from the joint because anabolic processes are unable to keep up with catabolism. Chronic occupational trauma to joints—such as that encountered by air-hammer workers—may result in osteoarthritis occurring in joints that usually are not involved in this disease, such as the wrists, elbows, and shoulders. The excessive secretion of growth hormone in patients with acromegaly is thought to be responsible for the thickening of synovial tissues and the overgrowth of joint cartilage that characterize the articular changes seen early in this disease. If acromegaly is untreated, marked degenerative changes will occur in joints. Because routine laboratory tests cannot detect the abnormalities, radiologic observation of changes occurring in joints still provides the most useful information for arriving at a diagnosis of degenerative joint disease.

135. The answer is A (1, 2, 3). *(Isselbacher, ed 9. p 1902.)* While it is suspected that metabolic defects, immunological defects, or both produce the chronic inflammation that results in the relapsing polychondritis syndrome, the pathogenesis of the disease remains unclear. The characteristic basophilic staining of normal cartilage that is revealed in hematoxylin and eosin preparations is lost in this disease. Inflammation in the cartilage of the nose and ears, which occurs in at least 80 percent of affected patients, produces the classic clinical signs of this condition. Both the ears and the nose become inflamed and painful, and progressive destruction of cartilage frequently results in severe disfigurement of the nose and drooping of the ears. The cartilaginous components of the external auditory meatus may be affected and progressive destruction may lead to a severe impairment of hearing. When relapsing polychondritis affects the upper respiratory tract and the bronchi, hoarseness may develop from involvement of the larynx. Reports have documented the fact that severe tracheal stenosis and even death from suffocation may occur if this major airway is destroyed. Recurrent pulmonary infections follow collapse of the cartilaginous tissue in the bronchi, leading to obstruction and stasis and subsequent bacterial overgrowth. The usual time of onset of this disease is in middle age and its natural history is characterized by periods of remission. Fortunately, the inflammation is sensitive to moderate doses of corticosteroids, which afford considerable relief for affected patients.

136. The answer is E (all). *(Isselbacher, ed 9. p 1879. Samter, ed 3. pp 1151-1156.)* Sjögren's syndrome consists of the triad of keratoconjunctivitis sicca, xerostomia, and a connective tissue disorder. The diagnosis is warranted when two of these three features are present. The connective tissue disease most commonly associated with the sicca complex is rheumatoid arthritis, but other diseases such as systemic lupus erythematosus, scleroderma, polymyositis, chronic active hepatitis, Waldenström's macroglobulinemia, pseudolymphoma, and malignant lymphoma also may be part of this complex. A group of patients afflicted with Sjögren's syndrome has been identified as having only the sicca complex (dry eyes and mouth). In this group, systemic complaints such as fatigue and arthralgias may be present.

137. The answer is C (2, 4). *(Beeson, ed 15. p 190. Isselbacher, ed 9. p 1874.)* Bouchard's nodes are bony enlargements around the proximal interphalangeal joints of the hand that occur in hypertrophic osteoarthritis. Necrotizing arteritis may arise in the course of rheumatoid arthritis and usually affects the skin, nervous system, and gastrointestinal tract but not the kidneys. In rheumatoid arthritis, subcutaneous nodules occur usually over the extensor surfaces in 10 to 20 percent of affected patients. Pulmonary manifestations also are associated with rheumatoid arthritis, including pleural effusions, pulmonary fibrosis, Caplan's syndrome, and pulmonary rheumatoid nodules.

138. The answer is C (2, 4). *(Isselbacher, ed 9. p 1875. McCarty, ed 9. pp 504-511.)* Rheumatoid factors are antibody molecules that react with antigenic determinants on other immunoglobulins. Most of these factors react equally well with aggregated gammaglobulin from both rabbit and human sources. In the conventional test for rheumatoid factor, aggregated gammaglobulin is attached to particles such as those of latex or bentonite and the ability of test sera to cause agglutination of these particles is determined. Diluted sera from approximately 70 percent of patients afflicted with rheumatoid arthritis will produce agglutination, whereas diluted sera from only about 5 percent of normal donors will do so. Rheumatoid factors of the IgG class also occur, but they are not easily detected by agglutination reactions.

139. The answer is E (all). *(Isselbacher, ed 9. p 1886.)* Behçet's disease is a multisystem disorder with a broad range of clinical features including (1) aphthous stomatitis, (2) genital ulcers, (3) iritis, (4) arthritis, (5) thrombophlebitis, (6) central nervous system lesions, (7) aseptic meningitis, and (8) peripheral neuropathy. The etiology of this disease is unknown. Histologic examination of involved tissues reveals vasculitis affecting arterioles and venules. In some affected patients, vasculitis may involve the vasa vasorum, resulting in aneurysms of large arteries and the aorta. One of the characteristic features of this disease is the development of sterile abscesses at the sites of tissue trauma such as hypodermic injection sites. This disease is most prevalent in the Middle East, but an increasing number of cases are being recognized in the western hemisphere.

140. The answer is B (1, 3). *(Isselbacher, ed 9. p 1894. McCarty, ed 9. pp 1161, 1172, 1177.)* Osteoarthritis is the most common form of joint disease in adults. When all age groups are considered, men and women are equally affected. The pathologic process is characterized by deterioration of articular cartilage and remodeling of subchondral bone to produce the characteristic picture of joint space narrowing, subchondral eburnation, and osteophyte formation. Joint trauma may initiate this disease even in young individuals.

141. The answer is D (4). *(Isselbacher, ed 9. p 2039. McCarty, ed 9. p 1020.)* Morton's metatarsalgia is a radicular pain that usually occurs as a consequence of pressure on the superficial branch of the plantar nerve as it passes between the fourth and fifth metatarsal heads; the disorder may result from lateral compression of the foot. The pain typically radiates up the leg or to the end of the toe. Prolonged irritation of the nerve at this area may lead to chronic neurologic changes and the development of a neuroma.

142. The answer is E (all). *(Isselbacher, ed 9. p 1897. McCarty, ed 9. pp 457, 491-500, 1161, 1172.)* Osteoarthritis has a predilection for weight-bearing joints and for joints subjected to repeated trauma. Thus, certain occupations predispose to osteoarthritis in particular joints, such as the knees and spine in coal miners, the shoulders in bus drivers, and the shoulders, elbows, and hands in pneumatic-tool workers. The lack of inflammation in affected joints and the absence of features of systemic disease help to distinguish osteoarthritis from rheumatoid arthritis. Osteoarthritis is usually associated with a normal sedimentation rate, noninflammatory synovial fluid that has a high viscosity, and little or no morning stiffness.

143. The answer is C (2, 4). *(Isselbacher, ed 9. pp 358-359.)* Procainamide and hydralazine are the drugs that are most likely to produce the "drug induced lupus syndrome." Patients who develop this syndrome produce antinuclear antibodies, as do patients with nondrug induced systemic lupus erythematosus. In both situations, positive fluorescent antibody tests that screen for all antinuclear antibodies will be positive. Antibodies that react with double-stranded or native DNA do not occur in patients suffering from drug induced lupus; the presence of these antibodies would suggest that nondrug induced lupus erythematosus is the true diagnosis. Antinative DNA antibodies are strongly associated with renal involvement in lupus erythematosus. Numerous nuclear and cytoplasmic cellular constituents act as antigens for patients with lupus erythematosus. Determination of the type of antibody that is produced and the titer of that antibody could be helpful in the diagnosis, and in establishing the prognosis and management of the disease. Renal involvement is extremely rare in drug-induced lupus syndromes;

moreover, patients with drug induced lupus erythematosus have a much lower frequency of central nervous system involvement than those with nondrug induced syndromes. In addition, complement levels usually are normal and antibodies to the drug itself do not occur.

144-148. The answers are: 144-B, 145-A, 146-E, 147-C. 148-D. *(Isselbacher, ed 9. p 1871.)* Examination of the synovial fluid may provide specific diagnostic information in infectious arthritis, gout, pseudogout, and in neoplastic diseases involving joints. Normal joint fluid is clear and colorless, has less than 200 white blood cells/mm^3 (most of which are mononuclear), and has a high viscosity. The viscosity, which correlates with the mucin clot, can be evaluated by observing a drop of synovial fluid released from a syringe. A normal viscosity will exhibit a string of fluid several inches long; fluid of diminished viscosity will behave like water.

Traumatic arthritis and osteoarthritis are usually associated with synovial fluid white blood cell counts of less than 2000/mm^3. In rheumatoid arthritis, Reiter's syndrome, gout, pseudogout, and other inflammatory forms of arthritis, synovial fluid white blood cell counts usually are in the range of 20,000 to 60,000/mm^3; in patients with pyogenic arthritis, white blood cell counts are frequently higher, especially when the infecting organisms are staphylococci or streptococci.

Synovial fluid complement levels may be helpful in distinguishing among some inflammatory forms of arthritis. Normal synovial fluid has a relatively low complement level in relation to the complement level in the blood because the large complement molecules do not easily penetrate the synovial membrane. When inflammation occurs, the synovium becomes more permeable, and complement components can then readily enter the joint space. In diseases such as rheumatoid arthritis, immune complexes are formed in synovial fluid. These complexes lead to complement activation; consequently, complement levels are decreased. Other inflammatory diseases, such as Reiter's syndrome, appear not to be associated with intra-articular complement consumption and are distinguished by having elevated complement levels.

In patients who have gout, synovial fluid examined by polarized light microscopy reveals negatively birefringent needle-shaped urate crystals; in pseudogout, smaller, more rhomboid-shaped crystals that exhibit weakly positive birefringence are seen.

Pulmonary Disease

DIRECTIONS: The question below contains five suggested answers. Choose the **one best** response.

149. All the following statements about *Mycoplasma pneumoniae* infections in adults are true EXCEPT that

(A) most infections are respiratory illnesses without pneumonia
(B) in the presence of pneumonia, cough is prominent though usually nonproductive
(C) unilateral consolidated infiltrates are common
(D) erythromycin eradicates the causative organism and alters the course of the illness
(E) tetracycline usually shortens the course of the disease

DIRECTIONS: Each question below contains four suggested answers of which **one** or **more** is correct. Choose the answer:

A	if	**1, 2, and 3**	are correct
B	if	**1 and 3**	are correct
C	if	**2 and 4**	are correct
D	if	**4**	is correct
E	if	**1, 2, 3, and 4**	are correct

150. Assisted ventilation using positive end-expiratory pressure (PEEP) is a recent and important development in treating respiratory failure. Correct statements concerning PEEP include which of the following?

(1) Its efficacy is attributed to its ability to increase functional residual capacity and maintain airway patency
(2) Water pressure levels of less than 10 cm do not lead to significant decreases in cardiac output
(3) Pneumothorax is an important and potentially fatal complication
(4) Its therapeutic benefit is enhanced by the utilization of Swan-Ganz catheterization

151. Effective early treatment for attacks of extrinsic asthma includes which of the following medications?

(1) Aminophylline
(2) Aerosolized corticosteroids
(3) Aerosolized beta-adrenergic agonists
(4) Cromolyn sodium

152. A 36-year-old woman with sarcoidosis has been managed conservatively for one year. During this period, despite radiographic evidence of extensive lung involvement, she has not had significant respiratory symptoms. She now complains of some exertional dyspnea associated with a cough and her physician reevaluates her case. Her chest x-ray shows little change. Pulmonary function tests are reported to show restrictive lung disease. Which of the following abnormalities would support the diagnosis of restrictive lung disease?

(1) A decrease in flow rates at midvital capacity compared to predicted values
(2) An increase in FEV_1/FVC ratio
(3) An increased functional residual capacity
(4) An increase in the alveolar-arterial oxygen tension difference

SUMMARY OF DIRECTIONS

A	B	C	D	E
1, 2, 3 only	1, 3 only	2, 4 only	4 only	All are correct

153. The maximum expiratory flow-volume curve is a new method of representing pulmonary function data. Correct statements concerning this method of representation include which of the following?

(1) The format contains all the data present in classic spirometry
(2) Obstruction is indicated by low flows only at low lung volumes
(3) The curve may be separated into effort-dependent and -independent portions
(4) Although restrictive defects may have a normal peak flow, the flow at the middle portion of the curve is reduced

154. Correct statements concerning the prognosis and clinical course of asthma include which of the following?

(1) Death from asthma is uncommon, with a death rate of approximately 1/300,000 persons
(2) About 45 percent of asthmatic children will still have symptomatic asthma 7-10 years after the initial diagnosis
(3) Sixty percent of patients whose asthma commences during adult life may expect to have little improvement in their disease as they grow older
(4) Throughout life there is a two-to-one, female-to-male preponderance

155. Correct statements regarding pulmonary function studies include which of the following?

(1) In emphysema, the diffusing capacity for carbon monoxide is abnormal
(2) In obstructive airway disease, the FEV_1/FVC ratio is reduced
(3) Chronic significant airway obstruction may be present despite a normal FEV_1
(4) In differentiating asthma from emphysema, the determination of residual volume is useful

156. Intermittent mandatory ventilation, a recent procedure in the treatment of patients in severe respiratory failure, is characterized by which of the following statements?

(1) It allows affected patients to regain coordination of their respiratory muscles
(2) It may be of help in weaning affected patients from respirators
(3) By allowing P_{CO_2} to "normalize," it helps to maintain cardiac output and cerebral blood flow
(4) It is especially useful in tachypneic, anxious patients

157. The risk of pulmonary thromboembolism is increased by which of the following factors?

(1) The postpartum state
(2) The use of birth control pills
(3) Venous insufficiency
(4) Primary pulmonary hypertension

Questions 158-159

A 28-year-old man enters the hospital with cough and fever. His admission x-ray is shown below. Acid-fast organisms, subsequently identified as *Mycobacterium tuberculosis,* are identified on a smear.

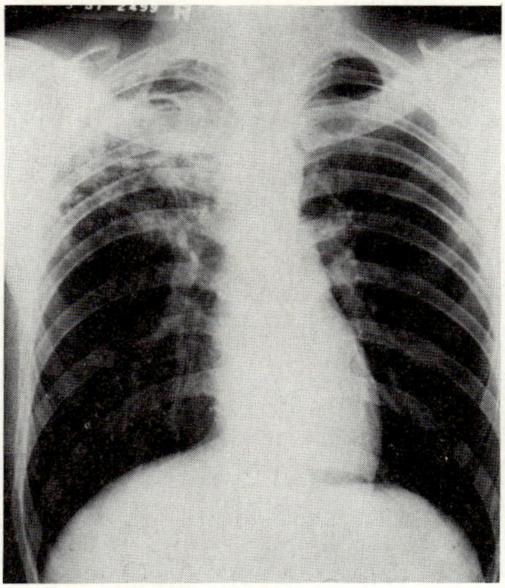

158. Correct statements regarding the pathophysiology of this patient's infection include which of the following?

(1) The initial exposure probably occurred at a time remote from the current symptoms
(2) The location of the current process probably resulted from inspiration of aerosolized droplets into the upper lobe
(3) Necrosis of the pulmonary lesion with cavity formation is a common complication of his condition
(4) Risk of infection to hospital staff will be reduced if the patient is kept on an open, well-ventilated ward

159. Currently acceptable management of the patient presented above would include which of the following measures?

(1) Isoniazid
(2) Rifampin
(3) Brief hospitalization during initiation of therapy
(4) Para-aminosalicylic acid

DIRECTIONS: The groups of questions below consist of lettered choices followed by several numbered items. For each numbered item select the **one** lettered choice with which it is **most** closely associated. Each lettered choice may be used once, more than once, or not at all.

Questions 160-165

Match the following.

(A) Asbestosis
(B) Silicosis
(C) Silo-filler's disease
(D) Pigeon-breeder's lung
(E) Byssinosis

160. When combined with cigarette smoking, predisposes affected patients to an increased risk of primary lung carcinoma

161. Caused by an antigen-antibody reaction within the lung; associated with dyspnea that is episodic or progressive or both

162. Caused by exposure to a toxic gas; associated with acute dyspnea and, occasionally, chronic fibrosis

163. Related to the development of malignant tumors of the pleura and peritoneum

164. Associated with nodular pulmonary infiltrates and hilar (eggshell) calcification

165. Associated with an increased risk of active tuberculosis

Questions 166-170

For each set of findings that follow, select the disease with which it is most likely to be associated.

(A) Asthma
(B) Rheumatoid arthritis
(C) α_1-antitrypsin deficiency
(D) Cystic fibrosis
(E) Bronchiectasis

166. High levels of lactic dehydrogenase in pleural effusions

167. Decreased synthesis of prostaglandins

168. Presence of the mucoid strain of *Pseudomonas aeruginosa*

169. Development of severe liver disease that is usually associated with, but may be independent of, lung disease

170. Progressive dyspnea, but very little coughing

Questions 171-175

For each statement that follows, select the histologic type of pulmonary neoplasm with which it is most clearly associated.

(A) Bronchial adenoma
(B) Adenocarcinoma
(C) Oat cell carcinoma
(D) Squamous cell carcinoma
(E) Bronchioloalveolar cell carcinoma

171. Almost always involves a history of smoking

172. Often presents with bronchorrhea and dyspnea

173. Surgery has not appreciably prolonged survival in affected patients

174. The lung cancer that is most radiosensitive

175. The lung cancer that is most likely to cavitate

Questions 176-180

For each clinical picture that follows, select the arterial blood gas and pH values with which it is most likely to be associated.

	pH	P_{O_2}	P_{CO_2}
(A)	7.54	75	28
(B)	7.15	78	92
(C)	7.06	36	95
(D)	7.30	58	44
(E)	7.39	48	54

176. A 30-year-old obese female bus driver develops sudden pleuritic left-sided chest pain and dyspnea

177. A 60-year-old heavy smoker has severe chronic bronchitis and peripheral edema and cyanosis

178. A 22-year-old drug-addicted individual is brought to the emergency room by friends who were unable to awaken him

179. A 62-year-old man who has chronic bronchitis and chest pain is given oxygen via mask in the ambulance en route to the hospital and becomes lethargic in the emergency room

180. A 20-year-old man brought to the emergency room is still wheezing 18 hours later despite vigorous therapy for episodic asthma

Pulmonary Disease
Answers

149. The answer is D. *(Isselbacher, ed 9. pp 759-761.)* Infections with *Mycoplasma pneumoniae* cause clinical pneumonia only in a minority of cases (less than 10 percent of infected military personnel; as many as 33 percent of infected family members); upper respiratory infections, including pharyngitis, bronchitis, and myringitis, predominate. Cough is often very bothersome and serves as a clue to diagnosis of this disease. Sputum production is scant. Although chest x-rays may reveal bilateral, hazy, basilar densities, evidence of unilateral infiltrates is the more common finding. Both erythromycin and tetracycline shorten the course of *Mycoplasma pneumoniae* infections, but the former may not eradicate the organism from the respiratory tract.

150. The answer is E (all). *(Isselbacher, ed 9. p 1277. Wayne, JAMA 236: 1394-1396, 1976.)* Positive end-expiratory pressure (PEEP) has found an important place in the therapy of severe respiratory failure, especially failure involving very low compliance and profound hypoxemia. The end-expiratory pressure serves to keep alveoli open, increasing functional residual capacity, and thus improving ventilation-perfusion relationships. The major complications of PEEP include pneumothorax and a decrease in venous return, with subsequent decrease in cardiac output. This change in cardiac output depends on the level of PEEP, intravascular volume, and lung compliance. Ten centimeters water pressure or more of PEEP may decrease cardiac output significantly and should not be administered to patients suffering from severe respiratory failure.

151. The answer is B (1, 3). *(Isselbacher, ed 9. pp 1208-1209.)* Aminophylline and beta-adrenergic agonists, both of which have proved effective in the treatment of asthma attacks, cause relaxation of smooth muscle by raising intracellular cyclic AMP concentration. Cromolyn sodium, of occasional use for prophylaxis in asthmatic patients, is delivered in a powdered form via a nebulizer. However, this substance may irritate the airways and lead to a worsening of cough and more severe bronchospasm. Parenterally administered corticosteroids are generally used in severe or persistent asthmatic episodes, but do not, in themselves, cause any immediate relaxation of bronchospasm. Nor do they immediately reverse the mucosal edema and the tenacity of the sputum often associated with an acute attack. Aerosolized corticosteroids have no place in the management of acute attacks of asthma. However, as a prophylactic measure, aerosolized corticosteroids such as beclomethasone should be added **after** an acute attack.

152. The answer is C (2, 4). *(Isselbacher, ed 9. pp 1196-1197, 1245.)* Sarcoidosis runs an unpredictable course. The lesions may spontaneously resolve or begin to organize and promote scarring that can disrupt the alveoli and produce restrictive lung disease. Evidence of such a course would be an indication for treatment with corticosteroids. Reliable information can be gained from pulmonary function tests. Restrictive lung disease is characterized by a decrease in total lung capacity. The associated decrease in the alveolar surface area, together with ventilation-perfusion inequality, diminishes the diffusing capacity and increases alveolar-arterial oxygen differences. The FEV_1 is supernormal early in the disease and well maintained even in advanced disease; the forced vital capacity falls, however. Thus, the FEV_1/FVC ratio tends to rise. Despite the fall in lung volume, flow rates over the middle portion of the FEV curve continue within the normal range. The functional residual capacity and the residual volume are increased in diseases, such as chronic bronchitis, that are characterized by increased airways resistance.

153. The answer is B (1, 3). *(Isselbacher, ed 9. p 1217.)* In the graphic display of pulmonary function data, the maximum expiratory flow-volume curve appears as a function of flow rate versus lung volume. Thus, flow at any given fraction of vital capacity may be determined. Because a time signal is incorporated, all the information contained in classic spirometry can be derived from the curve. In addition, the curve can be divided into two portions: an effort-independent mid-flow portion, and an effort-dependent initial (peak flow) and terminal portion. The effort-independent mid-flow is determined by compliance and small airways resistance. Flow during this portion of the curve increases as compliance falls and thus increases in restrictive disease. Obstructive diseases are manifested by low flow rates at high or normal lung volumes, as well as at low.

154. The answer is A (1, 2, 3). *(Isselbacher, ed 9. pp 1203, 1210.)* Owing to improvement in therapy, death from asthma is much less common than in the past. According to United States statistics gathered in 1973, nearly 2000 deaths from asthma were reported from all age groups in a one year period. Among patients between 5 years and 34 years of age, there were 250 deaths. In this age group, it is unlikely that other causes of death would have been confused with asthma. Thus the data are probably reliable. Calculations from these data yield a mortality rate for asthma of approximately 1/300,000 persons. Asthma is one of the more common diseases in the United States. It is estimated that 3 percent of the population of the United States, at some stage, suffer from reversible airways obstruction. Asthma occurs worldwide with an approximately equal frequency, except among West Africans, Eskimos, and American Indians, in whom it is uncommon. The natural course of asthma in children is better understood than in adults. Follow-up studies of children with asthma have revealed that ten years after the initial diagnosis, between 26 and 78 percent of affected patients will still be experiencing symptomatic episodes; the mean incidence for the persistence of clinically significant asthma is 46 percent. In contrast to adults, however, there is a tendency for children who continue to have asthma to experience less severe symptoms; only 19 percent of these patients continue with episodes that cause severe respiratory distress. In adults, it is unusual for asthma that develops in middle or later life to ameliorate spontaneously. Indeed, less than 20 percent of adults will become free of asthma and only 40 percent can expect improvement with less frequent and less clinically significant attacks in later years.

155. The answer is A (1, 2, 3). *(Bates, ed 2. pp 122, 147, 197. Isselbacher, ed 9. pp 1197-1198.)* Pulmonary function testing has become important in the diagnosis and assessment of severity of many acute and chronic pulmonary diseases. For instance, a decrease in the FEV_1/FVC ratio is important in diagnosing obstructive airways disease. In a patient who has a decrease in FEV_1, the ratio may be of use in separating obstructive from restrictive disease. Significant airway obstruction also may exist in the presence of a normal FEV_1 especially if the obstruction is localized to small (less than 2 mm diameter) airways. Determination of mid-expiratory flow rates using oxygen and helium are useful in diagnosing obstruction in these "small" airways. Since the residual volume is elevated in both asthma and emphysema, this index would not help to differentiate the two disorders. Because of parenchymal destruction in emphysema, the diffusing capacity is decreased.

156. The answer is A (1, 2, 3). *(Downs, Chest 64:331-335, 1973. Isselbacher, ed 9. p 1282.)* For patients suffering from severe respiratory failure, intermittent mandatory ventilation (IMV) has been of benefit in allowing them to use their own respiratory musculature while receiving mechanical ventilatory assistance. This procedure gradually prepares patients' ventilatory musculature and central control mechanisms for unassisted ventilation. However, injudicious use of IMV may actually lead to unnecessarily prolonged ventilatory support, and it is not necessary in all cases of respiratory deficit. IMV should be restricted to patients who are difficult to wean from respirators, who require ventilatory support for prolonged periods, or who have significant neurologic disorders like amyotrophic lateral sclerosis and myasthenia gravis. In agitated, tachypneic patients, the ventilator-delivered breaths may be ill-timed, leading to less effective ventilation and diminished pulmonary status. If such patients are adequately sedated, proper ventilation may effectively be delivered by standard controlled ventilation.

157. The answer is A (1, 2, 3). *(Isselbacher, ed 9. pp 1249-1254.)* Pulmonary emboli are found in disorders associated with hypercoagulability, venous abnormalities, and venous stasis. Venous stasis is exemplified in the postpartum period, and venous wall changes and alterations in coagulability are among the estrogen-mediated effects associated with birth control pills. Pulmonary emboli are not prominent features of primary pulmonary hypertension.

158. The answer is B (1, 3). *(Isselbacher, ed 9. pp 701-702.)* The patient described in the question has postprimary tuberculosis. The causative organism is initially inhaled by droplet aerosol into the lower lobes where ventilation is high. A primary, usually asymptomatic, infection ensues. Organisms are spread subsequently by hematogenous dissemination to other foci and grow best in those areas with a high oxygen tension, such as the upper lobe. Necrosis is part of the characteristic tissue reaction to infection. Symptomatic disease may then occur at these distant locations later in life. As the organism spreads by droplet aerosol, isolation of the patient becomes mandatory, preferably in a room with ultraviolet radiation.

159. The answer is A (1, 2, 3). *(Bobrowitz, Ann Rev Respir Dis 109:548-553, 1974. Isselbacher, ed 9. pp 707-710.)* The treatment of tuberculosis was revolutionized by the advent of chemotherapy, resulting in mass closures of tuberculosis sanitariums. Currently, the drug combination of choice for the treatment of tuberculosis is isoniazid and rifampin, provided there is no evidence that the infective organisms may be resistant to isoniazid. In the United States, this is not likely to be a problem, but patients who are infected with mycobacteria in the Philippines, Mexico, or Southeast Asia may have a form that is resistant to isoniazid. Although there is little to choose between the isoniazid-rifampin regimen and that of isoniazid and ethambutol, the latter would be the combination of choice in a patient suspected of having abnormal liver function. Hospitalization in association with the isoniazid-rifampin therapy can be brief and, in many cases, omitted completely, for although organisms may continue to be shed, they are noninfectious by approximately the second week of treatment. Rifampin is never used as a single agent owing to the rapid emergence of organisms resistant to this drug. Retreatment of resistant cases remains a difficult matter and requires a new combination of drugs. In such instances, it is desirable to use rifampin and isoniazid in combination with pyrazinamide and streptomycin. Para-aminosalicylic acid is no longer used as initial therapy for tuberculosis because of the multiple adverse reactions to this drug. Streptomycin is not needed except in therapy of multiple large cavities in which tubercle bacilli are thought to be numerous.

160-165. The answers are: 160-A, 161-D, 162-C, 163-A, 164-B, 165-B. *(Isselbacher, ed 9. pp 1212, 1218, 1220.)* Occupational lung disease may result from a variety of environmental conditions. Asbestos exposure for even short periods (less than two years) can produce an increased risk of lung carcinoma in smokers; longer exposure and a long latent period (10 to 20 years) usually are necessary, however, for the development of pleural and peritoneal involvement, which may take the form of pleural calcification and pleuroperitoneal malignancy.

Pigeon-breeder's disease involves an antigen-antibody reaction in the lung that is caused by exposure to pigeon antigens in pigeon droppings. The disease may present as an acute syndrome, or chronically as idiopathic fibrosis.

Silo-filler's disease, resulting from exposure to nitrogen dioxide liberated from silage, causes direct pulmonary injury. Repeated exposure to the gas may cause fibrosis.

Silicosis, which is seen in miners, sandblasters, and others exposed to silica, produces a nodular pattern on x-ray; eggshell calcification of hilar nodes is strongly suggestive of the disease. Progressive fibrosis can result, despite removal of affected patients from the silica dust environment. Massive nodules may form, accompanied by cavitation. Patients who have silicosis and are exposed to tuberculosis have a higher risk than persons without silicosis of developing the active form of tuberculosis; lifetime isoniazid therapy is currently advocated.

166-170. The answers are: 166-B, 167-A, 168-D, 169-C, 170-C. *(Isselbacher, ed 9. pp 1201, 1204, 1233, 1488. Mathiason, J Allergy Clin Immunol 64:669-674, 1979. Stennis, Clin Allergy 6:119-129, 1976.)* Pleural effusions are not unusual in patients with rheumatoid arthritis. A history of pleurodynia that would suggest an antecedent inflammatory pleuritis is not always obtained, but characteristically the pleural fluid, which is sterile, will contain a high level of lactic dehydrogenase and a low glucose concentration. Other pulmonary phenomena associated with rheumatoid arthritis include diffuse interstitial fibrosis and the occurrence of individual or clustered nodules in the lung parenchyma.

Asthma is frequently associated with bronchiolitis and immediate hypersensitivity reactions, but it should be kept in mind that exercise and intolerance to certain anti-inflammatory agents also are common triggering mechanisms for reversible airways obstruction. Fifteen percent of patients with asthma will experience bronchospasm shortly after the ingestion of aspirin or indomethacin, but not sodium salicylate. Other compounds that can produce the same effect, such as tartrazine yellow, the food coloring agent found in many drugs and as a coloring additive in over 200 food products, may be extremely difficult to avoid. Recent evidence suggests that in such patients these compounds are able to block cyclooxygenase activity needed to facilitate the reduction of arachidonic acid to prostaglandins. In the absence of this pathway, increased amounts of slow-reacting substance of anaphylaxis are produced.

The fatality rate for patients with cystic fibrosis is lower today than in previous years; currently, the average life span of patients afflicted with this disease is 19 years. Chronic lung infections, however, are almost universal. The most common and difficult to treat of such infections is caused by the mucoid strain of *Pseudomonas aeruginosa.* It is doubtful whether any form of antibiotic combination is effective in such patients. Distressing and chronic coughing is one of the major problems of patients with cystic fibrosis. Liver disease, particularly biliary cirrhosis, may develop in patients afflicted with *Pseudomonas aeruginosa* infections and about three percent of these patients present with portal hypertension.

The incidence of liver disease associated with a deficiency of α_1-antitrypsin is much higher than with *Pseudomonas aeruginosa* infections. Indeed, it is estimated that 15 percent of all chronic liver disease is associated with this deficiency. Panacinar emphysema with very little coughing is the predominant feature of the lung involvement.

171-175. The answers are: 171-D, 172-E, 173-C, 174-C, 175-D. *(Isselbacher, ed 9. pp 1259-1264.)* The incidence of carcinoma of the lung has increased steadily since 1900. Squamous cell carcinoma, the most common histologic type, is closely asociated with a history of cigarette smoking. The risk of lung cancer is twenty times greater in individuals who smoke one pack a day than in nonsmokers. Smoking is also known to increase the incidence of lung cancer in individuals exposed to asbestos well beyond the rate associated with exposure to asbestos alone. Symptoms from squamous cell carcinoma appear earlier than the symptoms of other lung tumors because the generally central location of the neoplasm causes bronchial obstruction.

Oat cell carcinoma accounts for less than 20 percent of primary lung carcinomas. It is radiosensitive, but because of a tendency to early metastasis, the prognosis for affected patients is poor. Several chemotherapeutic regimens, including immunotherapy, are currently being evaluated in patients who have oat cell carcinoma. Survival has not been improved by resectional surgery.

Bronchioloalveolar cell carcinoma is uncommon; when extensive, this tumor may lead to profuse bronchorrhea and death from hypoxia and respiratory failure. This type of carcinoma may present as a local mass lesion or a diffuse bilateral infiltrate.

Although adenocarcinoma may cavitate, squamous cell carcinoma is much more likely to do so. Adenocarcinoma may develop peripherally and thus become manifest as metastatic disease, the chest lesion remaining clinically "silent."

Adenocarcinoma may arise from old scars such as those of healed tuberculosis or interstitial fibrosis.

Bronchial adenoma is an uncommon neoplasm. It grows very slowly and may produce various symptoms like hemoptysis, bronchial obstruction, and carcinoid syndrome.

176-180. The answers are: 176-A, 177-E, 178-C, 179-B, 180-D. *(Bates, ed 2. pp 130, 452-454. Isselbacher, ed 9. p 1198.)* The blood gas values associated with pulmonary embolism may vary tremendously. It is important to note that hypoxemia need not be present, as illustrated in the laboratory values accompanying the question.

In severe chronic lung disease, the presence of hypercapnia leads to a compensatory increase in serum bicarbonate. Thus, significant hypercapnia may be present with an arterial pH close to normal.

Acute respiratory acidosis may occur secondary to respiratory depression after drug overdose. Hypoventilation is associated with hypoxia, hypercapnia, and severe, uncompensated acidosis.

In the presence of long-standing lung disease, respiration may become regulated by hypoxia rather than by altered carbon dioxide tension and arterial pH, as in normal individuals. Thus, the unmonitored administration of oxygen may lead to respiratory suppression, as in the patient described in the question.

In asthmatic episodes, significant hypoxia is not uncommon. After 18 hours, an affected patient's strength may be waning so that eucapnia or hypercapnia may be present rather than the hypocapnia characteristic of respiratory alkalosis; this normalization of P_{CO_2} signals the onset of respiratory failure.

Cardiology

DIRECTIONS: Each question below contains five suggested answers. Choose the **one best** response to each question.

181. Congenital complete heart block is characterized by all the following statements EXCEPT that

(A) the conduction defect usually lies above the bundle of His
(B) most affected patients require pacemakers before 12 years of age
(C) affected patients have a normal cardiac output
(D) the neck veins of affected patients demonstrate intermittent cannon *a* waves
(E) the resting pulse of affected patients is usually above 40/minute

182. The earliest electrocardiographic indication of acute pericarditis is

(A) concave upward ST-segment elevation
(B) convex upward ST-segment elevation
(C) ST-segment depression
(D) T-wave inversions
(E) tall peaked T waves

183. Each of the following statements regarding the effect of digitalis is true EXCEPT that

(A) in the patient who does not have congestive failure, it increases cardiac output
(B) in the patient who does not have congestive failure, it increases peripheral vascular resistance
(C) in the patient who does not have congestive failure, it increases myocardial oxygen consumption
(D) in the patient who has congestive failure, mitral stenosis, and normal sinus rhythm, it is of limited benefit
(E) in the patient who has cardiogenic shock, it is of little value

184. Endocarditis is commonly associated with all the following congenital cardiac lesions EXCEPT

(A) ventricular septal defect
(B) pulmonic stenosis
(C) atrial septal defect
(D) tetralogy of Fallot
(E) patent ductus arteriosus

185. A 75-year-old woman suffering from an acute anterior wall myocardial infarction is admitted to a coronary care unit. An ECG monitor strip, obtained six hours after admission, discloses the rhythm illustrated below. This rhythm probably represents

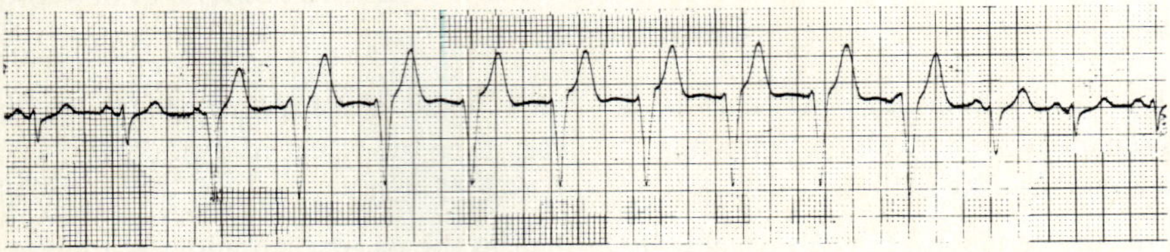

(A) rate-dependent left bundle branch block
(B) rate-dependent right bundle branch block
(C) complete heart block
(D) accelerated idioventricular rhythm
(E) junctional rhythm

---

186. A 53-year-old man suffering from an acute inferior wall myocardial infarction is admitted to the coronary care unit. Physical examination reveals a pulse of 68/minute, blood pressure of 150/90 mm Hg, and no evidence of congestive heart failure. Four hours later, he develops a sinus bradycardia at a rate of 42/minute. The patient remains asymptomatic and his blood pressure is 120/80 mm Hg. The patient should now receive

(A) careful observation
(B) intravenous atropine sulfate, 0.6 mg
(C) intravenous isoproterenol
(D) intravenous epinephrine
(E) a temporary transvenous pacemaker

187. On the fifth day of hospitalization for his first myocardial infarction, a 56-year-old man develops mitral regurgitation and left-sided heart failure. Despite treatment with inotropic agents and diuretics over the next two weeks, the failure steadily worsens. Although it seems that the patient may need surgery, his physicians are anxious to control him medically for at least another two weeks. In view of evidence that left ventricular afterload is contributing to this man's heart failure, it has been decided to administer a vasodilator, of which the most suitable in this case would be

(A) nitroglycerine
(B) isosorbide dinitrate
(C) phentolamine
(D) hydralazine
(E) trimethaphan

188. The prolapsed mitral valve syndrome is characterized by all the following EXCEPT

(A) single or multiple systolic clicks
(B) ST-segment depression and T-wave inversion in leads II, III, and aVF
(C) frequent arrhythmias
(D) high incidence of response to digitalis
(E) low incidence of sudden death

189. Single probe, unidirectional echocardiography has become a major tool in the noninvasive diagnosis of heart disease. The LEAST accurate statement concerning echocardiography is which of the following?

(A) It is useful in the diagnosis of idiopathic hypertrophic subaortic stenosis
(B) Patients with a prolapsing mitral valve have a characteristic echocardiogram
(C) Ultrasonic evaluation of the motion of the pulmonary valves is valuable in the diagnosis of pulmonary incompetence in the absence of an audible murmur
(D) Echocardiography supplies a reliable noninvasive method for distinguishing pericardial effusion from a dilated heart
(E) Recent advances in echocardiography have been particularly useful in defining the anatomic defects in infants with cyanotic heart disease

190. Radioisotopic examination of the cardiovascular system is proving to be increasingly useful. All the following statements concerning this technique are true EXCEPT that

(A) the injection of macroaggregated ^{131}I-labeled albumin with subsequent scanning of the lung fields is valuable in the detection of pulmonary emboli
(B) coronary artery disease produces poor myocardial perfusion that can be safely detected in resting patients using thallium 201 (^{201}Tl), which allows ischemic areas to be recognized as "cold spots"
(C) the bone-imaging radiopharmaceutical, technetium 99m stannous pyrophosphate (^{99m}TcPYP), concentrates in acutely damaged myocardial tissue to produce a "hot spot" image 12 to 24 hours after myocardial infarction
(D) measurements of ventricular performance that are independent of geometric assumptions can be made during initial passage of technetium 99m (^{99m}Tc)
(E) a totally normal perfusion scan (^{99m}TcPYP) 24 to 48 hours after the onset of pain occurs in less than 5 percent of patients with acute myocardial infarction

191. All the following statements regarding myxomas are true EXCEPT that they

(A) are the most common primary cardiac tumor
(B) are commonly associated with atrial fibrillation
(C) may present as a peripheral embolus
(D) may cause mitral regurgitation
(E) may produce systemic symptoms such as fever, weight loss, or arthralgias

192. Type IV hyperlipoproteinemia is associated with all the following conditions EXCEPT

(A) glucose intolerance in 50 percent of affected patients
(B) elevated endogenous triglycerides
(C) generally normal cholesterol levels
(D) coronary artery disease
(E) frequent occurrence of eruptive xanthomas

193. Idiopathic hypertrophic subaortic stenosis is characterized by all the following statements EXCEPT that

(A) the carotid pulse of affected patients reveals a slow upstroke
(B) the associated murmur increases in a standing position
(C) a prominent fourth heart sound frequently occurs
(D) mitral regurgitation is present in 50 percent of affected patients
(E) propranolol is useful for treating affected patients who have dyspnea or light-headedness

194. A 40-year-old man with a five-year history of essential hypertension and diabetes, managed by alpha methyldopa and oral hypoglycemic agents respectively, is brought to the emergency room. The patient reports that for 24 hours he has had a severe frontal headache, increasing confusion, nausea and, most recently, decreased visual acuity. His systolic blood pressure is too high for measurement with the standard sphygmomanometer. His diastolic blood pressure is 190 mm Hg. The physician should immediately institute which of the following therapies?

(A) Intravenous administration of methyldopa, 500 mg in 200 ml of 5 percent dextrose over 30 minutes
(B) Simultaneous intravenous administration of glucose, 30 g and hydralazine, 10 mg
(C) An intravenous push of diazoxide, 150 mg followed by a repeat dose if the diastolic blood pressure does not fall within two minutes
(D) An intravenous bolus of 0.5 μg/kg of body weight of nitroprusside
(E) Simultaneous intravenous administration of furosemide, 100 mg and trimethaphan, 15 mg

195. A 54-year-old man is admitted to the coronary care unit for symptoms of retrosternal chest pressure, nausea, and intense diaphoresis. An electrocardiogram on admission reveals ST-segment elevation in leads V_1 to V_4. An electrocardiogram obtained the following day is shown below. Which of the following steps should next be taken in the management of this patient?

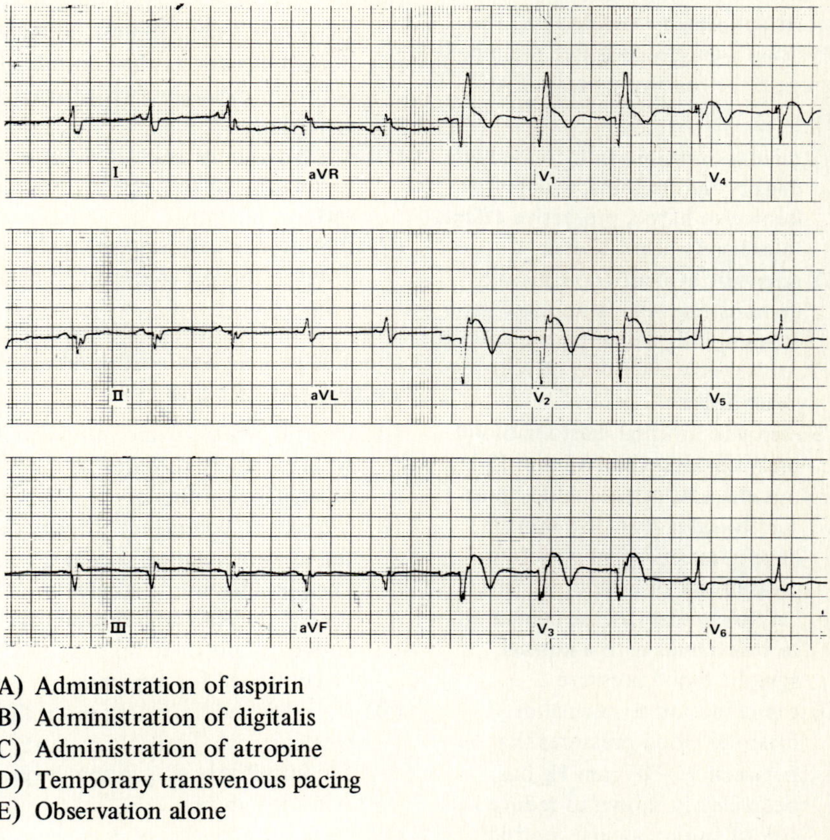

(A) Administration of aspirin
(B) Administration of digitalis
(C) Administration of atropine
(D) Temporary transvenous pacing
(E) Observation alone

196. A 45-year-old white male accountant is recovering from his first anterior myocardial infarction. As part of a program to control this patient's ischemic heart disease, his doctor discusses with the patient certain risk factors and how to avoid them. The physician would be justified in emphasizing all the following points EXCEPT that

(A) regular exercise can increase high density lipoproteins, which are known to have a protective effect in ischemic heart disease
(B) scientific evidence conclusively demonstrates that stopping cigarette smoking decreases the risk of further complications of ischemic heart disease
(C) men with normal diastolic blood pressures (less than 82 mm Hg) but elevated systolic blood pressure (greater than 158 mm Hg) have in excess of a two-fold increased risk of developing severe cardiovascular disease compared to individuals with a normal systolic blood pressure
(D) the reduction to normal of diastolic blood pressures that lie between 95-105 mm Hg has been clearly shown to reduce the risk of cardiovascular morbidity
(E) a family history of xanthomata is associated with an increased risk of ischemic heart disease

197. All the following statements regarding coarctation of the aorta are ture EXCEPT that

(A) affected patients may complain of leg pain or fatigue
(B) it rarely produces symptoms of congestive heart failure in infancy
(C) it has a higher risk than normal of occurring in patients with Turner's syndrome
(D) it is commonly associated with aortic stenosis due to a bicuspid valve
(E) the lesion usually appears just distal to the left subclavian artery

198. All the following statements about acute deep venous thrombosis are true EXCEPT that

(A) heparin, administered intravenously, is currently accepted as the most effective therapy
(B) it is safe to commence therapy on the basis of findings obtained with Doppler ultrasound studies
(C) for isolated calf area thrombosis, anticoagulant treatment should be continued for 4-6 weeks
(D) a ^{125}I-labeled fibrinogen test is the best currently available method for definitively diagnosing deep vein thrombosis
(E) there is a high risk of deep vein thrombosis in malignancy involving the pancreas, the lung, and the gastrointestinal tract

199. The rhythm strip displayed below reveals normal sinus rhythm with

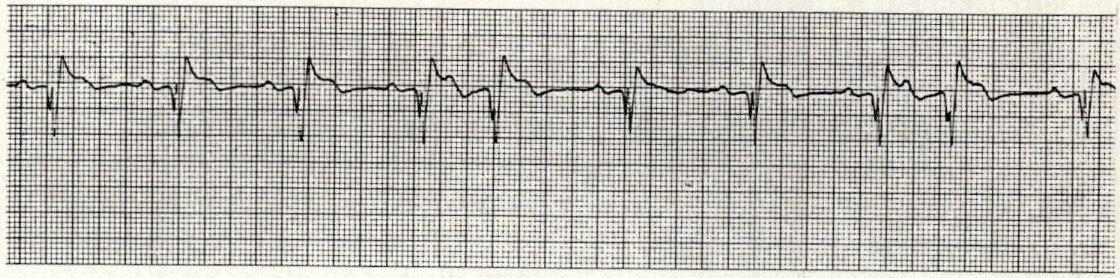

(A) periods of atrioventricular dissociation
(B) periods of Wenckebach atrioventricular block
(C) atrial premature contractions
(D) junctional premature contractions
(E) ventricular premature contractions

---

200. The rhythm strip (lead II) shown below was obtained from a patient who had severe obstructive lung disease. The strip most closely resembles which of the following arrhythmias?

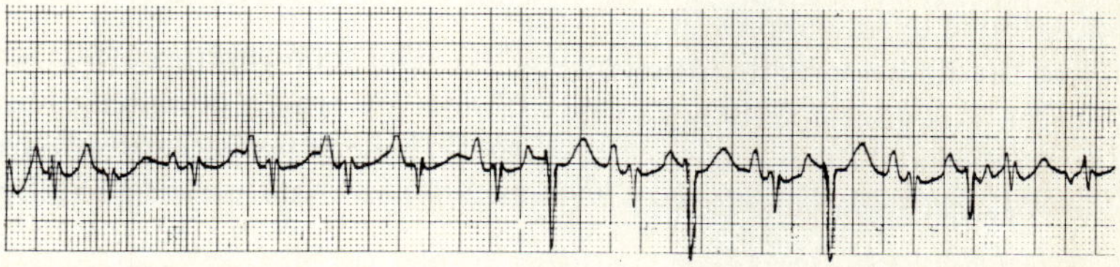

(A) Atrial flutter with varying atrioventricular block
(B) Sinus tachycardia with premature atrial contractions
(C) Sinus tachycardia with premature ventricular contractions
(D) Atrioventricular dissociation
(E) Multifocal atrial tachycardia

201. A 61-year-old man with mild hypertension but no symptoms is found to have a pulsating mass in the midepigastrium. Continuous ultrasound B scanning confirms the diagnosis of an aneurysm of the abdominal aorta. All the following statements about this disease are true EXCEPT that

(A) there is a 15-20 percent chance that the aneurysm will rupture if the diameter is less than 6 cm
(B) the mortality rate associated with surgery for a ruptured abdominal aortic aneurysm is 50 percent
(C) in the absence of other cardiovascular disease, surgery for small aneurysms (4-6 cm in diameter) is not indicated
(D) ultrasound examination will disclose the diameter of the aneurysm
(E) prognosis is most closely linked to the presence of other arteriosclerotic cardiovascular disease

202. Coronary bypass surgery results in relief or improvement of angina in what percent of affected patients?

(A) Less than 30 percent
(B) 30 to 40 percent
(C) 50 to 60 percent
(D) 80 to 90 percent
(E) 90 to 100 percent

203. A 25-year-old woman is seen by a cardiologist for evaluation of a heart murmur. The patient has no history of rheumatic fever and states that the murmur has been present for many years. Examination reveals normal first and second heart sounds and no evidence of cardiomegaly. A grade II/VI systolic ejection murmur is heard in the second right intercostal space. In addition, an ejection sound is heard over the aortic area. The most likely diagnosis is

(A) idiopathic hypertrophic subaortic stenosis
(B) subvalvular aortic stenosis
(C) valvular aortic stenosis
(D) supravalvular aortic stenosis
(E) functional or innocent murmur

204. The main pharmacologic action of nitroglycerin in producing a therapeutic benefit for patients who have angina pectoris is the drug's ability to

(A) dilate coronary arteries
(B) dilate peripheral arteries
(C) dilate systemic veins
(D) increase coronary blood flow by increasing heart rate
(E) slow heart rate and thus myocardial oxygen consumption

205. All the following statements about abnormalities in cardiac rhythm or rate are true EXCEPT that

(A) the treatment of sinus bradycardia (a rate less than 60/min) following myocardial infarction is mandatory if an affected patient is experiencing ventricular premature beats occurring at a rate of three or more per minute
(B) ventricular tachycardia occurring after myocardial infarction can be initially treated with lidocaine if an affected patient is not in heart failure
(C) digoxin is not contraindicated in the management of cardiac failure associated with ventricular tachycardia
(D) anticoagulation therapy is of little use in patients with atrial fibrillation who suffer thromboemboli following elective reversion to sinus rhythm
(E) quinidine should never be used in patients with atrial flutter without the prior or concomitant administration of digoxin or propranolol

206. A syphilitic aneurysm of the aorta is most likely to occur at which of the following sites?

(A) Ascending aorta
(B) Aortic arch
(C) Descending thoracic aorta
(D) Abdominal aorta
(E) Bifurcation of the iliac arteries

207. An 18-year-old man is involved in a street fight during which he sustains a severe knife wound to the chest. As a consequence of this injury, bleeding occurs into his pericardial cavity. He is placed on broad-spectrum antibiotic coverage that includes ampicillin and gentamicin. He makes a good recovery over the following month but three months after the incident he suddenly becomes ill with a fever of 39.6°C (103.3°F). The symptoms and signs consist of pericarditis, pleuritis, and pneumonitis. In the three days that follow, the patient develops arthralgias, pericardial effusion, and leukocytosis. The most likely diagnosis of this condition is

(A) serum sickness induced by ampicillin
(B) rheumatoid arthritis
(C) Dressler's syndrome
(D) acute idiopathic pericarditis
(E) acute bacterial endocarditis

208. Paradoxic splitting of the second heart sound may occur in association with each of the following cardiovascular disorders EXCEPT

(A) aortic stenosis
(B) right bundle branch block
(C) left bundle branch block
(D) left ventricular ischemia
(E) hypertension

209. A 40-year-old woman who had rheumatic fever at ten years of age has had a heart murmur for the past 15 years. Over the past three years she has noted progressive dyspnea on exertion, orthopnea, and fatigue. She is presently unable to do even light housework without developing shortness of breath and fatigue. Physical examination reveals a loud first heart sound and opening snap that is very close to the second heart sound. There is a grade III/VI mid-diastolic rumble at the cardiac apex with presystolic accentuation. Cardiac catheterization reveals pure mitral stenosis with a calculated valve area of 0.8 cm^2. No mitral regurgitation is present. Management of this patient should consist of

(A) penicillin prophylaxis
(B) administration of anticoagulants
(C) digitalization
(D) mitral valve commissurotomy
(E) mitral valve replacement

210. Each of the following statements regarding ventricular aneurysms is true EXCEPT that

(A) they should be suspected in the presence of a persistent ST-segment elevation following a myocardial infarction
(B) they are more common with anterior than inferior wall myocardial infarctions
(C) affected patients have an increased risk of cardiac rupture
(D) recurrent arterial emboli may be the presenting sign
(E) the diagnosis may be suggested by the x-ray finding of calcium in the cardiac border

211. All the following statements regarding aortic regurgitation are true EXCEPT that

(A) 75 percent of patients with pure aortic incompetence are male
(B) 15 percent of patients with a ventricular septal defect will have associated aortic incompetence
(C) aortic regurgitation may occur in patients with congenital bicuspid aortic valves
(D) symptomatic regurgitation in patients with rheumatic valve disease usually develops within one year of the initial endocarditis
(E) in chronic, severe aortic incompetence, the first symptom is often an uncomfortable awareness of the heart beat

212. The organism most commonly involved in right-sided endocarditis is

(A) *Streptococcus faecalis*
(B) *Streptococcus viridans*
(C) *Staphylococcus aureus*
(D) a gram-negative species
(E) *Candida albicans*

213. Each of the following statements regarding corrected transposition of the great vessels is true EXCEPT that

(A) it is commonly associated with ventricular septal defects
(B) it involves a left-sided atrioventricular valve that has three cusps
(C) it is associated with a loud and palpable second heart sound in the second left intercostal space
(D) it commonly involves first, second, and third degree heart block
(E) affected patients frequently complain of dyspnea and fatigue

214. The electrocardiogram displayed below is most compatible with which of the following diagnoses?

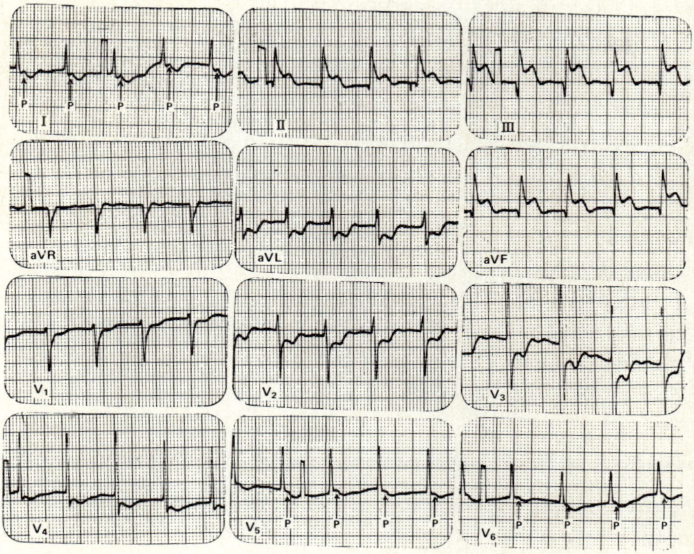

(A) Acute pericarditis with nodal tachycardia
(B) Acute anterior wall myocardial infarction with nodal tachycardia
(C) Acute inferior wall myocardial infarction with nodal tachycardia
(D) Acute inferior wall myocardial infarction with complete heart block
(E) Acute anterolateral myocardial infarction with nodal tachycardia

215. The rhythm strip displayed below demonstrates

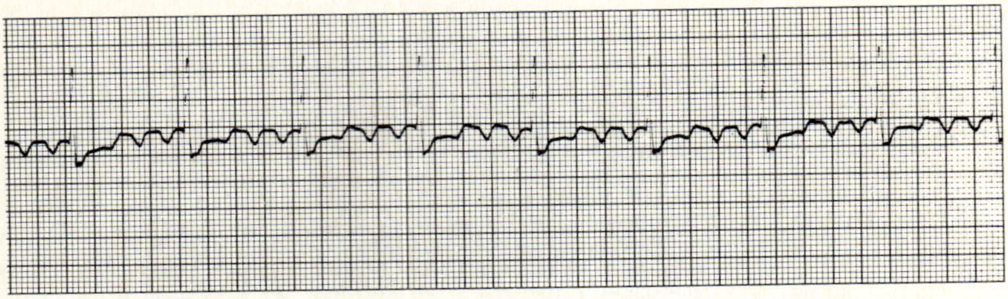

(A) normal sinus rhythm
(B) junctional rhythm
(C) atrial flutter with 4:1 atrioventricular block
(D) paroxysmal atrial tachycardia with 2:1 atrioventricular block
(E) complete heart block
with 2:1 atrioventricular block
(E) complete heart block

216. The rhythm strip shown below demonstrates which of the following arrhythmias?

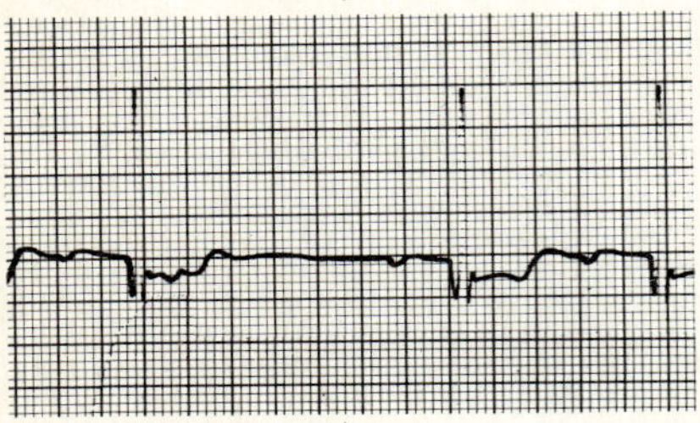

(A) Sinus arrhythmia
(B) Sinus arrest
(C) Sinoatrial block
(D) Wenckebach atrioventricular block
(E) Blocked atrial premature contraction

217. A 45-year-old man is admitted to the hospital for an acute anteroseptal myocardial infarction. Physical examination reveals a blood pressure of 150/100 mm Hg and pulse of 100/minute. The lung fields are clear and cardiac examination reveals only an S_4 gallop. Two days following admission, the patient develops severe shortness of breath. Blood pressure is 100/70 mm Hg, pulse 120/minute, and respiratory rate 32/minute. There are apical rales bilaterally. A grade III/VI systolic murmur is present at the lower left sternal border and both S_3 and S_4 gallops are present. The P_{O_2} is 70 mm Hg. The most likely diagnosis is

(A) pericardial effusion with tamponade
(B) papillary muscle dysfunction
(C) ruptured papillary muscle
(D) rupture of the interventricular septum
(E) acute pulmonary embolus

218. A 65-year-old man complains of chest pain, shortness of breath, and syncope. He has a long history of a heart murmur but was asymptomatic until one year ago when he noted retrosternal chest pain occurring on exertion but relieved by rest. The chest pains have continued, and he has noted exertional dyspnea for the past several months. On two occasions following heavy exertion, the patient passed out for several seconds. Physical examination reveals a blood pressure of 110/80 mm Hg and pulse of 50/minute. The carotid upstroke is markedly delayed; there is a palpable systolic thrill. Lung fields reveal rales in both bases. The point of maximum intensity is in the fifth intercostal space, mid-clavicular line. There is a prominent left ventricular heave. The first heart sound is soft and aortic closure is decreased. A grade IV/VI harsh, late-peaking systolic murmur is heard over the aortic area. Third and fourth heart sounds are present at the apex. The electrocardiogram reveals sinus bradycardia and left ventricular hypertrophy. The chest x-ray shows cardiomegaly with congestive heart failure. The most appropriate measure in the management of this patient would be

(A) stress testing
(B) cardiac catheterization
(C) oral propranolol and long-acting nitrates
(D) diuretics and digitalis
(E) a permanent pacemaker

219. A 23-year-old woman with no previous history of cardiac disease develops symptoms and signs of acute bacterial endocarditis with mitral incompetence one week after an abortion. *Streptococcus faecalis* is grown in blood cultures. The most appropriate treatment for this patient would be

(A) mitral valve replacement followed by six weeks of antibiotic therapy
(B) parenteral administration of ampicillin, 12 grams daily for four weeks
(C) parenteral administration of penicillin G, 24 million units daily for six weeks
(D) parenteral administration of penicillin G, 24 million units per day, and gentamicin, 4 mg/kg daily for four weeks
(E) parenteral administration of vancomycin, 1 g daily for four weeks with streptomycin, 1 g daily added to the protocol for the first two weeks

220. A 25-year-old woman is seen by her physician because of progressive dyspnea, fatigue, and syncope on exertion. She has no history of rheumatic fever or heart murmur. The patient was in excellent health until six months ago when her symptoms developed; they have since become progressively worse. Physical examination reveals a well-developed, well-nourished, acyanotic woman who experiences mild respiratory distress at rest. The jugular pulse reveals large *a* waves. There is a prominent right ventricular heave. A palpable pulmonic closure is present. A grade III/VI systolic ejection murmur is heard at the left second intercostal space. A grade I/VI blowing, holosystolic murmur is also noted at the lower left sternal border. The pulmonic closure is loud but splits normally with inspiration. The electrocardiogram reveals right ventricular hypertrophy. A chest x-ray shows dilatation of the main pulmonary arteries with decreased vascularity in the outer one-third of the lung fields. The most likely diagnosis is which of the following?

(A) Atrial septal defect
(B) Ventricular septal defect
(C) Congenital pulmonic stenosis
(D) Tetralogy of Fallot
(E) Primary pulmonary hypertension

221. All the following statements about rheumatic fever are true EXCEPT that

(A) the vast majority of patients with carditis do not have symptoms referable to the heart
(B) approximately 75 percent of attacks of acute rheumatic fever subside within six weeks
(C) a diagnosis of rheumatic fever without serologic evidence of a recent streptococcal infection is unwarranted
(D) there are no data from controlled clinical trials to suggest that corticosteroids are useful in the treatment of rheumatic carditis
(E) the best antibiotic regimen to prevent recurrence of Group A streptococcal infection is the administration of benzathine penicillin, 1.2 million units monthly

222. Each of the following statements regarding the effects of alcohol on the heart is true EXCEPT that

(A) alcoholic cardiomyopathy is usually not associated with alcoholic cirrhosis
(B) patients afflicted with alcoholic cardiomyopathy may have premature ventricular contractions or sinus tachycardia
(C) patients who have alcoholic cardiomyopathy commonly develop mural thrombi
(D) in normal patients alcohol decreases cardiac output
(E) the most important therapy for alcoholic cardiomyopathy is abstinence from alcohol

223. A 50-year-old man with a long history of heavy cigarette smoking is admitted to a coronary care unit for an acute inferior wall myocardial infarction. Blood pressure on admission is 140/90 mm Hg, pulse rate 80/minute, and respiratory rate 16/minute. Cardiac examination reveals a loud S_4 gallop only. The patient is given intravenous furosemide, 40 mg, and has a profound diuresis. Twelve hours later, his blood pressure is 80/60 mm Hg, pulse rate 88/minute, and he complains of retrosternal chest pain. A Swan-Ganz pulmonary artery catheter is passed and the patient's pulmonary capillary wedge pressure is 4 mm Hg. The most appropriate immediate therapy would be

(A) infusion of normal saline
(B) infusion of norepinephrine
(C) infusion of dopamine
(D) intravenous furosemide, 40 mg
(E) intravenous digitalis

224. A 45-year-old asymptomatic airline pilot is subjected to exercise-induced cardiac stress tests as part of a biannual physical examination. At the end of a quite strenuous exercise test (heart rate greater than 150/minute), he develops a 3 mm ST-segment depression in leads V_1 to V_4. However, he has no pain or other symptoms. There is no family history of early ischemic heart disease or hypertension. The patient has normal lipid studies. The advice you would give to this patient should be which of the following?

(A) The risk of sudden myocardial ischemia is too high to allow you to continue as a commercial pilot
(B) You should have coronary angiography to determine the condition of your coronary vessels
(C) You should have the test repeated in a month; if it is still positive, you should stop flying and have coronary angiography
(D) You can continue to fly safely only if you receive anticoagulants and take long-acting drugs to dilate your coronary blood vessels
(E) Your electrocardiographic changes are without significance and correlate poorly with sudden death and other complications of heart disease

225. An 82-year-old woman is admitted to the coronary care unit because of episodes of syncope. The patient suddenly becomes unresponsive, and the rhythm strip displayed below is obtained. Pulse and blood pressure are unobtainable. The most appropriate immediate therapy would be to administer

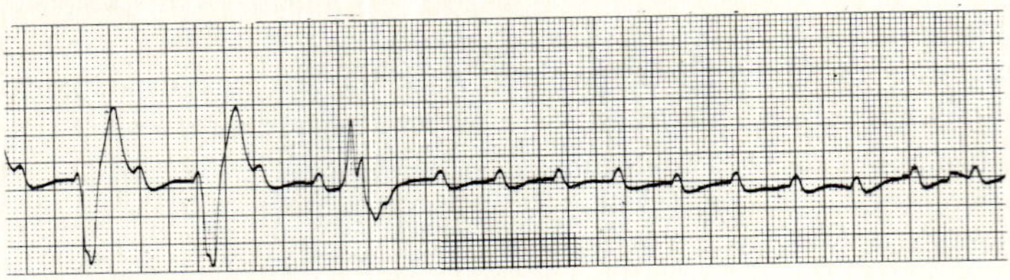

(A) isoproterenol by infusion
(B) norepinephrine by infusion
(C) intravenous lidocaine, 50 mg bolus
(D) intravenous atropine, 1 mg
(E) intracardiac epinephrine

---

226. The electrocardiogram displayed below reveals which of the following abnormalities?

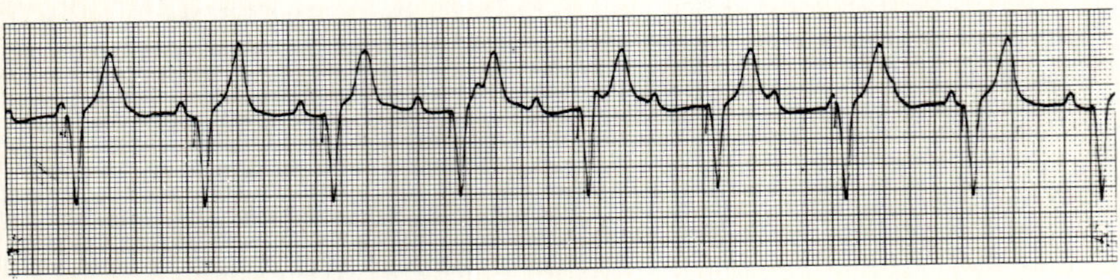

(A) Atrioventricular (AV) dissociation
(B) Paced rhythm with 100 percent capture
(C) Complete heart block
(D) Mobitz I second degree (Wenckebach) AV block
(E) Normal sinus rhythm with first degree AV block and blocked atrial premature contractions

227. The electrocardiogram displayed below reveals which of the following patterns?

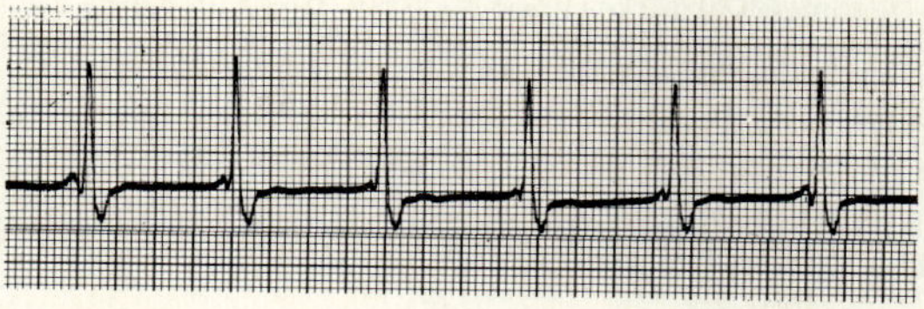

(A) Normal sinus rhythm
(B) Junctional or nodal rhythm
(C) Idioventricular rhythm
(D) Complete heart block
(E) Atrioventricular dissociation

DIRECTIONS: The groups of questions below consist of lettered choices followed by several numbered items. For each numbered item select the **one** lettered choice with which it is **most** closely associated. Each lettered choice may be used once, more than once, or not at all.

Questions 228-231

For each electrolyte abnormality that follows, select the electrocardiographic picture with which it is most commonly associated.

(A) No known electrocardiographic abnormalities
(B) Prolonged Q-T interval
(C) Short Q-T interval
(D) Widened QRS complex
(E) Prominent U waves

228. Hypokalemia

229. Hyperkalemia

230. Hypocalcemia

231. Hyponatremia

Questions 232-235

For each clinical situation listed below, select the drug or drug related toxicity with which it is most closely associated

(A) Furosemide
(B) Atropine
(C) Propranolol
(D) Digitalis toxicity
(E) None of the above

232. Chronic obstructive lung disease

233. Severe pericardial effusion

234. Ventricular tachycardia in a patient receiving quinidine

235. Gynecomastia

Questions 236-239

For each of the following drugs, select the mechanism of action with which it is most closely identified.

(A) Decreased renin release
(B) Peripheral vasodilatation
(C) Reduction of intravascular volume
(D) Depletion of norepinephrine from peripheral nerves
(E) Decreased central nervous system sympathetic stimulation

236. Hydralazine

237. Clonidine

238. Guanethidine

239. Propranolol

Questions 240-242

Match the following.

(A) Bronchiectasis
(B) Coarctation of the aorta
(C) Ventricular septal defect
(D) Homocystinuria
(E) None of the above

240. Dextrocardia

241. Aortic and pulmonary artery dilatation

242. Hyperextensible joints

Questions 243-247

A normal jugular venous pulse wave in relation to first and second heart sounds is displayed below. For each cardiac phenomenon described, select the segment of the venous pulse wave with which it is most likely to be associated.

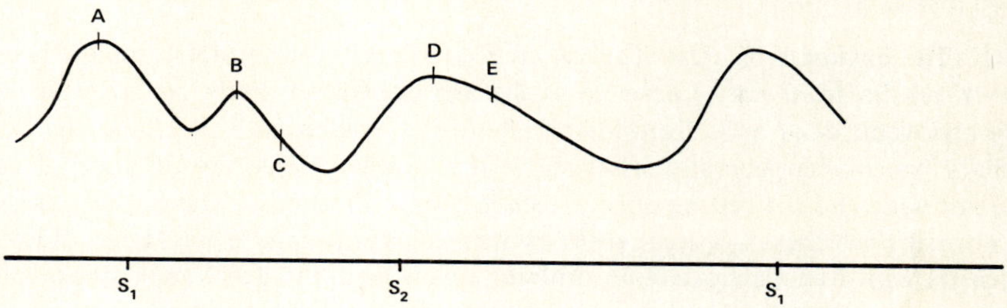

243. Atrial contraction

244. Filling of right atrium while tricuspid valve is closed

245. Opening of tricuspid valve

246. Bulging of tricuspid valve into right atrium

247. S_4 gallop

Questions 248-250

For each congenital heart defect that follows, select the murmur with which it is most characteristically associated.

(A) Murmur of aortic stenosis
(B) Murmur of mitral regurgitation
(C) Murmur of pulmonic stenosis
(D) Murmur of tricuspid regurgitation
(E) Murmur of aortic regurgitation

248. Ebstein's anomaly

249. Anomalous left coronary artery arising from the pulmonary artery

250. Ostium secundum atrial septal defect

Questions 251-253

For each cardiac disorder that follows, select the clinical finding with which it is most closely associated.

(A) Sharp *y* descent in jugular pulse tracing
(B) Mid-diastolic rumble at apex
(C) Large *v* waves in jugular pulse tracing
(D) Slow *y* descent in jugular pulse tracing
(E) Prominent *c* waves in jugular pulse tracing

251. Tricuspid stenosis

252. Aortic regurgitation

253. Constrictive pericarditis

Cardiology Answers

181. The answer is B. *(Isselbacher, ed 9. p 1061.)* Congenital complete heart block results from either absence of the atrioventricular node or separation of the atrioventricular node from the bundle of His by fibrous tissue. Since the subsidiary pacemaker generally arises above the bundle of His, the QRS complexes are not wide and the resting pulse is usually 40 to 60/minute. The cardiac output is normal since there is a compensatory increase in stroke volume. Many affected patients can even participate in athletic events without developing symptoms. Cannon *a* waves in the jugular pulse are seen with complete heart block from any cause and result from intermittent contraction of the atrium against a closed tricuspid valve.

182. The answer is A. *(Isselbacher, ed 9. pp 1150-1154.)* The electrocardiogram of acute pericarditis differs in several respects from that seen in acute myocardial infarction. ST-segment elevation in pericarditis tends to be concave upwards, whereas in infarction the ST segments are convex upwards. In addition, pericarditis incurs T-wave inversion as a later sign that appears only after the ST segments have returned to baseline; but in acute myocardial infarction, the T waves may invert while the ST segments are still elevated. Yet another differentiating point between these lesions is that with the ST-segment elevation of acute myocardial infarction in one ECG lead, there is usually reciprocal ST-segment depression in other leads. The ST-segment elevation of pericarditis does not have reciprocal ST-segment depressions.

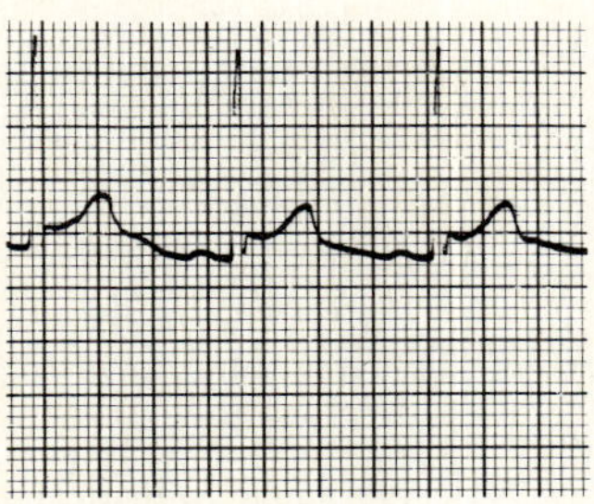

Pericarditis

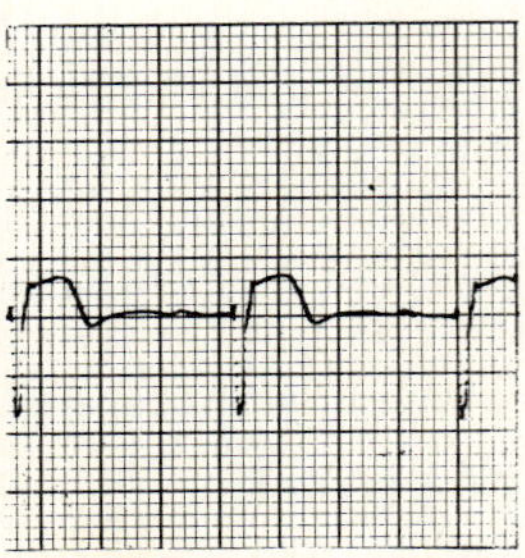

Acute Myocardial Infarction

183. The answer is A. *(Isselbacher, ed 9. p 1065. Mason, pp 323-326.)* Administration of digitalis to a patient who has congestive heart failure increases cardiac output. In a patient who does not have congestive failure, digitalis increases contractility but not cardiac output because the increase in contractility is offset by an increase in peripheral vascular resistance, which is a direct effect of the drug. In patients who have actual mechanical obstruction (mitral or aortic stenosis), digitalis is of limited benefit. However, in patients who have mitral stenosis with rapid atrial fibrillation, digitalis is of great benefit in slowing the ventricular rate and allowing more time for emptying of the left atrium. The main determinant of myocardial oxygen consumption is wall tension, which increases in cardiac failure. In a patient who has cardiac failure, digitalis reduces both wall tension and myocardial oxygen needs; in a normal patient, it increases contractility and myocardial oxygen requirements. Digitalis offers little to the patient suffering cardiogenic shock because the primary defect is a tremendous loss of muscle tissue.

184. The answer is C. *(Isselbacher, ed 9. pp 1075-1089. Weinstein, Prog Cardiovasc Dis 16:250, 1973.)* Atrial septal defects are rarely involved in endocarditis probably because there is no large pressure gradient across the defect. Significant pressure gradients created by other congenital cardiac lesions result in turbulence, which appears to be one of the predisposing factors for the deposition of fibrin and bacteria.

185. The answer is D. *(Isselbacher, ed 9. p 1130. Lichstein, Am J Med 58:197-198, 1975.)* The ECG strip presented in the question demonstrates normal sinus rhythm with a period of accelerated idioventricular rhythm (AIVR). AIVR may arise from increased automaticity or occur as an escape rhythm, and usually is seen either after acute myocardial infarction or in digitalis intoxication. On the ECG, the rate of the AIVR is slightly faster than that of the first two sinus beats. Beats numbered 3 and 12 represent fusion beats since the QRS configuration is intermediate between that of the sinus beats and those of the AIVR. Characteristics of this arrhythmia are the wide, bizarre complexes resembling premature ventricular contractions, the presence of fusion beats, and a rate of 55 to 125/minute. Rate-dependent left or right bundle branch block is accompanied by widening of the QRS complex but each complex is preceded by a constant P-R interval. In complete heart block, P waves are independent of the QRS complexes and occur at a rate faster than the QRS complexes. Junctional rhythms most commonly occur at rates of 40 to 60/minute and the QRS complexes are usually normal in configuration.

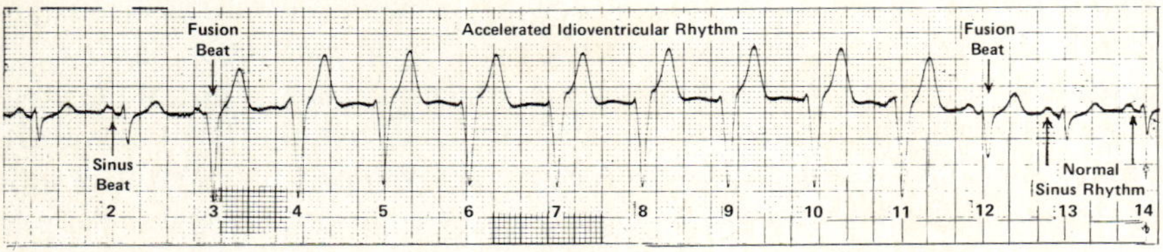

186. The answer is A. *(Isselbacher, ed 9. p 395. Rotman, Circulation 45:706, 1972.)* Sinus bradycardia is common following acute myocardial infarction involving the inferior wall. It results from a combination of ischemia to the sinus node and increased parasympathetic activity. In the clinical situation presented in the question, in which the patient is asymptomatic and normotensive, no immediate therapy is indicated. Should the bradycardia cause hemodynamic compromise, intravenous atropine should be given.

187. The answer is D. *(Isselbacher, ed 9. p 1043.)* Many compensatory changes occur in the heart and vascular bed of patients experiencing heart failure. One such mechanism involves the active constriction of peripheral vessels. This constriction results in persistent tension in the myocardium of the left ventricle (left ventricular afterload). If cardiac function is already impaired, this additional factor may significantly worsen the situation by reducing cardiac output and further increasing myocardial consumption of oxygen. A major advance in the treatment of severe heart failure has been the development of drugs that can dilate the peripheral vessels, thus reducing vessel wall obstruction to left ventricular ejection. The various vasodilators that are available have different hemodynamic effects, loci, and durations of action. The modes of administration also differ. The ideal vasodilating drug would be administered orally and have a sustained effect for at least six hours. Some vasodilators, such as the alpha-adrenergic blocking agents and hydralazine, affect the arterial bed while others, such as nitroglycerin, only affect resistance in the venous circulation. Hydralazine is an ideal choice for the patient who needs long-term treatment and vasodilation of the arterial circulation. Nitroglycerine has a short lived effect on the venous system. Isosorbide dinitrate affects the same vessels but is longer acting than nitroglycerin. Phentolamine, which works on arterial beds, lasts for minutes only and must be given by continuous intravenous infusion. The same objections apply to trimethaphan. Nitroprusside, which affects both venous and arterial beds, is ideal for the management of acute heart failure. It is effective for only minutes, however, and must be given by continuous intravenous infusion.

188. The answer is D. *(Isselbacher, ed 9. p 1103. Reduto, Postgrad Med 60:172-174, 1976.)* The prolapsed mitral valve syndrome, known also as the "floppy" mitral valve syndrome, is characterized by prolapse of one or both mitral leaflets into the left atrium during systole. The associated click or clicks tend to occur in midsystole and are thought to result from the tensing of the chordae tendineae as the mitral leaflets move into the left atrium. Classically, there is a late systolic murmur resulting from mitral regurgitation. While the electrocardiogram often is normal in these patients, there may be ST-segment and T-wave abnormalities in the inferior leads. Affected patients often complain of palpitations and atrial or ventricular arrhythmias. Echocardiography has proved to be very effective in establishing the diagnosis of the prolapsed mitral valve syndrome. The drug of choice for the arrhythmias associated with the syndrome is the beta-blocking agent, propranolol. Digitalis is ineffective in most cases. A very small percentage of these patients die suddenly, presumably from arrhythmias.

189. The answer is C. *(Isselbacher, ed 9. p 1016.)* Echocardiography has assumed great importance in the investigation of cardiac disease. The technique can supply accurate information about all areas of the heart, with the exception of the pulmonary valve. The movements of the cusps of the mitral valve, however, are easily visualized. It is possible to diagnose mitral stenosis even in the absence of a diastolic murmur, a situation that commonly occurs when patients are suffering from severe pulmonary hypertension associated with a decreased cardiac output. The aortic valve, as well as the area around the valve, are well visualized. Hypertrophic subaortic stenosis is readily diagnosed by echocardiography. Left atrial myxomas and congestive cardiomyopathy also can be detected by this technique, which provides valuable information on cardiac disturbances in congenital disorders, situations in which noninvasive techniques are of particular value. Echocardiography currently provides the most accurate way of diagnosing and assessing the severity of pericardial effusions. The echocardiograph technique is based on the excitation of ceramic compounds with the subsequent generation of short, high frequency electrical signals that provide inaudible ultrasonic pulses. The ultrasonic wave forms are reflected at the point where they pass from tissue of one density into tissue of another density. These echoes, which are transmitted and received at a rate of more than 1000 impulses per second, are amplified and displayed on an oscilloscope.

190. The answer is B. *(Isselbacher, ed 9. p 1012.)* Myocardial ischemia in patients with coronary artery disease is associated with areas of poor blood flow in which damage to heart muscle occurs. Radioisotope scanning with the radionuclide thallium 201 (^{201}Tl) can often detect these areas. After an intravenous injection of the isotope, which has a half-life of 72 hours, myocardial distribution of isotope, proportional to myocardial blood flow, will rapidly occur. Less of the radionuclide will accumulate in areas of ischemia, giving rise to cold spots on the scan. To utilize the full potential of the technique, a stress test is often needed because patients with preinfarctional ischemic disease often have normal scans at rest. With exercise, myocardial oxygen consumption will increase and normal areas will receive an appropriate compensatory increase in blood flow. Those areas perfused by diseased coronary vessels will receive relatively less tracer. The most efficacious time to inject the isotope is when exercise produces either chest pain or electrocardiographic changes consistent with ischemia.

191. The answer is B. *(Isselbacher, ed 9. pp 1147-1148.)* Myxomas most commonly involve the left atrium, are usually pedunculated and friable, and frequently embolize. The tumor may move across the mitral or tricuspid valves causing blockage, thus mimicking mitral or tricuspid stenosis. Myxomas also may prolapse on their pedicles into the ventricle, thus preventing closure of the mitral or tricuspid valves. They should always be considered in a patient who has changing murmurs, intermittent episodes of syncope, or congestive failure, and in the patient with an unexplained peripheral arterial embolus. It is significant that myxomas may also cause systemic symptoms such as fever, weight loss, or arthralgias; the affected patient's laboratory values may be abnormal, including an elevated sedimentation rate, white blood cell count, or serum globulin. Echocardiography is useful in demonstrating the presence of myxomas.

192. The answer is E. *(Isselbacher, ed 9. pp 507-518. Levy, Curr Probl Cardiol 1:23-24, 1976.)* Type IV hyperlipoproteinemia is characterized by normal to mildly elevated cholesterol levels and an increase in endogenous triglycerides. Very low density lipoproteins will be elevated, since they consist mainly of triglycerides derived endogenously from small bowel and liver. It appears that type IV hyperlipoproteinemia is associated with an increased risk of coronary artery disease and is commonly associated with glucose intolerance and hyperuricemia. Xanthomas can occur but are unusual.

193. The answer is A. *(Isselbacher, ed 9. p 1144.)* Idiopathic hypertrophic subaortic stenosis (IHSS) is characterized by thickening of the muscular interventricular septum resulting in obstruction to left ventricular ejection of blood during ventricular systole. The typical murmur is a systolic ejection murmur along the left sternal border. Any maneuver that increases left ventricular volume will decrease the obstruction and murmur. Conversely, standing, which causes venous pooling in the lower extremities, will decrease ventricular volume and thus cause the obstruction and murmur to increase. The arterial pulse has a typical brisk upstroke and may display two palpable peaks in the pulse wave. A loud fourth heart sound is common and results from the atrium attempting to eject blood into a thick, noncompliant ventricle. The thick septum associated with IHSS, by displacing the anterior leaflet of the mitral valve, causes mitral regurgitation in 50 percent of affected patients. Propranolol, by decreasing the contractility of the heart, may relieve the obstruction to left ventricular ejection, thus relieving symptoms like dyspnea on exertion, chest pain, or light-headedness.

194. The answer is C. *(Isselbacher, ed 9. pp 1177-1178.)* Prior to recent advances in the treatment of malignant hypertension, the mean survival time was only two years. The patient described in the question exhibits the symptoms of malignant hypertension. The rapidly progressive nature of his symptoms presents a danger of convulsions and imminent loss of vision. The condition is a true medical emergency, and calls for immediately reducing the diastolic pressure in the direction of, but not below, 90 mm Hg. If the hypertensive state is less advanced than that described in the question, methyldopa, reserpine, or hydralazine may be used. However, all these drugs must be given by constant infusion and are relatively slow-acting (20 minutes to three hours). Diazoxide is the drug of choice, even in diabetic persons (anti-insulin effects of this drug are not a problem in the short term). It can be given as an intravenous bolus and usually works immediately. Some physicians recommend 300 mg as a starting dose, but it is more customary to give 150 mg initially and administer a second bolus only if the response is unsatisfactory. Nitroprusside and trimethaphan act in less than a minute but must be given by continuous infusion; the effect of these drugs lasts for only two to five minutes. Diazoxide brings the blood pressure down instantly, the effect lasting from four to 12 hours. Malignant hypertension may present with symptoms and signs of hypertensive encephalopathy. Some patients who had died in a hypertensive crisis exhibited multiple small cerebral thrombi at autopsy. Dilatation of cerebral arteries and generalized arteriolar fibrinoid necrosis contribute to the associated symptoms and signs. The cerebral arteries dilate because the normal autoregulation of cerebral blood flow decompensates secondary to the markedly elevated arterial pressure. Cerebral blood flow is thus excessive and encephalopathy follows. The average age of onset of malignant hypertension is 40 years; men are predominantly affected.

195. The answer is D. *(Chung, ed 2. pp 595-599. Isselbacher, ed 9. pp 1006-1007.)* The electrocardiogram shown in the question reveals an evolving anteroseptal myocardial infarction. There is ST-segment elevation in leads V_1 to V_4 with Q waves present in leads V_1 to V_3. Right bundle branch block (RBBB) is present with QRS duration of 0.12 second and terminal, wide S waves in leads I, aVL, and V_6. The classic rSR′ of RBBB is not seen since the initial r wave in V_1 has been replaced with a Q wave as a result of the anterior infarction. The electrocardiogram also reveals marked left axis deviation consistent with a left anterior hemiblock. Since both the right bundle and the anterior division of the left bundle are damaged as a result of the infarction, conduction to the ventricles is dependent solely on the posterior division of the left bundle. In the presence of an acute anteroseptal myocardial infarction, temporary transvenous pacing is indicated for the patient involved as a prophylactic measure to avert complete heart block.

196. The answer is D. *(Isselbacher, ed 9. p 1167.)* To date, reduction of excessive cardiovascular morbidity has been demonstrated clearly only in patients whose diastolic pressures had exceeded 105 mm Hg. There is a growing concensus among cardiologists, however, that the diastolic pressure should be kept at, or below, 90 mm Hg. Excellent evidence now suggests that high density lipoproteins, which can absorb 20 percent of the total plasma cholesterol, protect against the development of atherosclerosis and, therefore, should be considered to be anti-risk factors. A decrease in cigarette smoking and the undertaking of regular exercise both raise the circulating level of high density lipoproteins. Epidemiological studies have conclusively demonstrated the benefit of stopping cigarette smoking, as well as the dangers of smoking. Elevations in systolic blood pressure, though less damaging than elevations in diastolic blood pressure, are definitely associated with an increased risk of cardiovascular disease.

197. The answer is B. *(Isselbacher, ed 9. p 1084.)* Coarctation of the aorta consists of a region of narrowed aorta; 95 percent of these lesions occur just distal to the left subclavian artery. Because of decreased blood flow to the lower extremities, affected patients may complain of leg fatigue or pain on exertion. A congenital bicuspid aortic valve occurs concomitantly with coarctation in approximately 50 percent of such individuals. Symptoms of congestive heart failure are common in infants who have coarctation, and usually appear in the first months of life. Patients afflicted with Turner's syndrome have a high incidence of aortic coarctation.

198. The answer is D. *(Isselbacher, ed 9. p 1187.)* Hospitalized patients undergoing prolonged bed rest are at risk of developing acute venous thrombosis. It is the most common vascular disorder encountered in hospitals. While the major and minor deep veins of the leg and pelvis are most frequently affected, thrombosis can occur at many sites. In addition to bed rest, predisposing factors that have been identified include (1) malignancy, especially that involving the pancreas, lung, and gastrointestinal tract, (2) postpartum period, (3) treatment with estrogen preparations including oral contraceptives, (4) disseminated intravascular coagulation, and (5) neuroparalysis of the upper or lower limbs. Occasionally, venous thrombosis will occur following trauma or bacterial infection. Clotting usually starts in the soleus plexus of veins and in the sinus of the venous valves. It is extremely difficult, if not impossible, to make a bedside diagnosis of acute venous thrombosis. Initial diagnoses must be confirmed independently before treatment can be started. The tests currently accepted as the most effective noninvasive diagnostic techniques are Doppler ultrasound and plethysmography. ^{125}I-labeled fibrinogen is useful only before clinical signs and symptoms develop. Its primary use is in patients thought to be at high risk for the development of venous thrombosis. If a thrombosis does occur, the radiation emitted by the isotope will allow precise localization of the problem. The currently accepted treatment of choice is intravenous heparin. Duration of therapy is dependent on the degree of involvement and whether or not pulmonary embolization is present. If a patient experiences pulmonary embolization, anticoagulant therapy with heparin must be started immediately and continued for at least 10 to 14 days, even longer if the patient is still thought to be at risk. It is currently recommended that patients be started on an oral anticoagulant before heparin is stopped, thus ensuring a smooth transition from one drug to another. Anticoagulants have no effect on thrombi, but they do prevent their extension and further thrombotic episodes. Anticoagulation with oral agents should be continued for three to six months if large vessels—such as the femoropopliteal or iliofemoral veins—have been involved, with or without pulmonary embolization. For isolated calf vein thrombosis, it is sufficient to use oral anticoagulants for four to six weeks.

199. The answer is C. *(Chung, ed 2. pp 98-101. Isselbacher, ed 9. p 1007.)* The rhythm strip shown below, and in the question, demonstrates normal sinus rhythm with two atrial premature contractions (beats numbered 5 and 9). Atrial premature contractions are characterized by P waves that occur earlier than the next sinus beat and differ in morphology form the P waves of the sinus beats. They may be conducted to the ventricles resulting in relatively normal-appearing QRS complexes or, if they occur during the refractory period of the ventricles, they may be blocked. In this situation, premature P waves would differ in morphology from the P waves of the sinus beats and no QRS complex would follow the P wave. Atrial premature contractions may occur singly or may result in atrial flutter, atrial fibrillation, or atrial tachycardia.

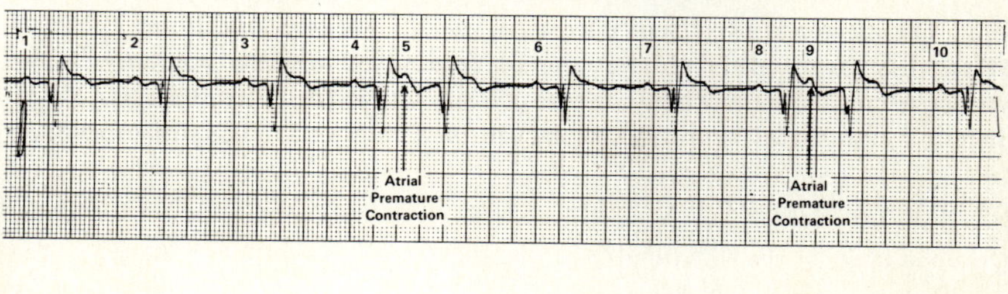

200. The answer is E. *(Chung, ed 2. pp 114-124. Isselbacher, ed 9. p 1056.)* Multifocal atrial tachycardia tends to occur in patients who have severe lung disease. It is characterized by varying P-wave morphology and P-R intervals. The rhythm strip shown below exhibits at least three different P-wave shapes. The beats numbered 8, 10, and 12 are probably aberrantly conducted, resulting in their more bizarre appearance. The presence of severe pulmonary disease in the patient from whom the strip was obtained is suggested by the tall, peaked P waves (P pulmonale).

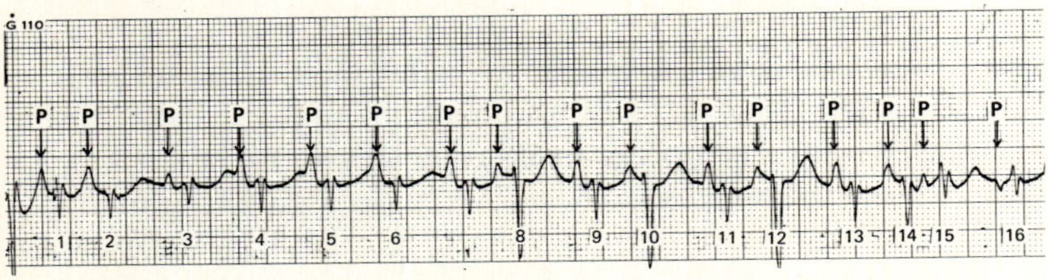

201. The answer is C. *(Isselbacher, ed 9. pp 1178-1179.)* Seventy-five percent of aortic aneurysms occur in the abdominal aorta just below the renal arteries. The majority of such aneurysms occur in men; the mean age of occurrence is 60. More than half the cases are associated with elevations in blood pressure. Most commonly the diagnosis is made on routine physical examination. Ultrasound is the noninvasive investigation of choice and will delineate the mass and provide the diameter of the aneurysm and the thickness of its walls. Small diameter aneurysms (less than 6 cm) present a 15-20 percent chance of rupture. However, as fatalities associated with this complication approximate 50 percent and the operative mortality for elective procedures of small diameter aneurysms is only 5 percent, it is prudent to recommend surgery for affected patients. Five-year survival rates for patients with aortic aneurysms without cardiovascular disease is 50 percent; with cardiovascular disease it is only 20 percent. In the presence of other cardiovascular disease, small diameter aneurysms may be followed by serial ultrasound examinations. Risks associated with surgery in these patients is substantial. Information on changes in the aneurysm provided by ultrasound examinations would be useful in making a decision on the necessity of surgery.

202. The answer is D. *(Isselbacher, ed 9. pp 1123-1124.)* Additional longitudinal studies are needed before it can be determined whether coronary bypass surgery decreases the mortality rate associated with ischemic heart disease. Nevertheless, a number of firm conclusions can be drawn on the basis of procedures that have been performed to date. Angina is relieved in 85 percent of affected patients, although many of them will still require postoperative drug therapy for best results. In most good hospitals, mortality associated with the operation itself is extremely low (approximately 1 percent) and the patency of the grafted vessels remains good in 70 to 80 percent of patients for at least two to three years following surgery. One problem hindering acceptance of the coronary bypass technique has been the inability to demonstrate significant hemodynamic improvement in left ventricular function after surgery. In deciding which patients to recommend for bypass surgery, it is useful to keep in mind that the mortality for patients with disease isolated to either the circumflex or right coronary artery is low, being very little different from that of age-matched controls. On the other hand, when the left or main coronary artery is involved, the mortality rate is extremely high and surgical intervention must be seriously considered.

203. The answer is C. *(Isselbacher, ed 9. pp 1085-1086.)* The patient discussed in the question probably has congenital aortic stenosis with a bicuspid aortic valve. An ejection sound is a useful clue to this diagnosis because it means that the murmur is generated by the valve leaflets that snap open in systole. Ejection sounds are high frequency sounds that follow the first heart sound and may originate on either the left or right side of the heart. They may result from ejection of blood into a dilated aorta or pulmonary artery as well as from the snapping open of a stenotic semilunar valve. Ejection sounds may be absent when calcification of the abnormal valve later in life prevents snapping open of the leaflets. Ejection sounds would not be present with subvalvular or supravalvular aortic stenosis or with idiopathic hypertrophic subaortic stenosis. In addition, the systolic ejection murmur of idiopathic hypertrophic subaortic stenosis tends to be maximal along the lower left sternal border.

204. The answer is C. *(Isselbacher, ed 9. p 1122. Mason, pp 350-353.)* Nitroglycerin relieves angina chiefly by dilating the systemic veins. By thus pooling the blood and diminishing venous return, nitroglycerin effectively decreases left ventricular size, wall tension, and myocardial oxygen consumption. (Wall tension is the greatest determinant of myocardial oxygen consumption.) To a lesser degree, nitroglycerin achieves anginal relief by dilatation of peripheral arterioles. This effect reduces resistance to ejection of blood and so, in a sense, decreases the work the heart must do in ejecting blood. In a patient who has coronary artery disease and atherosclerotic vessels, it is unlikely that nitroglycerin exerts any significant effect upon the coronary circulation itself.

205. The answer is D. *(Isselbacher, ed 9. pp 1056, 1130-1131.)* In patients with atrial fibrillation, especially those with mitral stenosis, thromboembolic complications are common. Thromboembolism is responsible for about 20 percent of deaths in patients with mitral stenosis. Long-term anticoagulation therapy has been shown to be advantageous in the treatment of these patients. Anticoagulants should be given for at least two weeks before attempting to reinstate sinus rhythm. Sinus bradycardia is dangerous when ventricular premature beats are present; the low sinus rate facilitates the development of ventricular tachycardia. However, there is no agreement as to the best treatment of sinus bradycardia itself in patients who have experienced myocardial infarction. Indeed, some studies suggest that sinus bradycardia is indicative of a favorable prognosis. Ventricular tachycardia is a serious problem—lidocaine may be tried as the therapy of first choice if the dysrhythmia occurs soon after infarction and the patient has no undue distress. If 100-200 mg of intravenous lidocaine do not control the dysrhythmia, electrical conversion should be attempted. Quinidine, by enhancing atrioventricular conduction, may enhance ventricular rates in patients with atrial flutter. Thus, there is a need for digoxin or propranolol in quinidine-treated patients with atrial flutter.

206. The answer is A. *(Hurst, ed 4. pp 1665-1666. Isselbacher, ed 9. pp 720, 1179.)* Aneurysms of the aorta from syphilis occur most commonly in the ascending aorta and least commonly in the descending thoracic and abdominal aorta. Calcification in the wall of the ascending aorta is frequently present. Aneurysm formation occurs 15 to 30 years following infection with syphilis. Syphilis may affect the cardiovascular system in several additional ways. Aortic valvular insufficiency is the most common complication of syphilitic aortitis. In addition, syphilis may involve the coronary ostia resulting in progressive occlusion and symptoms of angina or myocardial infarction.

207. The answer is C. *(Isselbacher, ed 9. p 1152.)* Dressler's syndrome may develop following the escape of blood into the pericardial cavity from a variety of causes (e.g., cardiac surgery, myocardial infarction, trauma to the heart from a nonpenetrating blow to the chest, perforation of the heart by a pacemaking catheter). The syndrome usually occurs two to four weeks following the cardiac injury but quite frequently appears after a lapse of months, even years. Relapses are very common. Symptoms of Dressler's syndrome include fever, pleuritis, pericarditis, pneumonitis, arthritis, and leukocytosis. The syndrome, which is thought to be a result of immunological sensitization to cardiac antigens presented to lymphocytes at the time of the injury, correlates with the presence of antimyocardial antibodies; the clinical picture associated with the syndrome resembles that seen with both viral and idiopathic pericarditis. In the patient presented in the question, the history of a knife wound helps to eliminate those entities as diagnostic possibilities. Often no treatment other than mild analgesics is needed, but the problem can be very serious and even fatal. Severe cases usually respond to corticosteroids. Rheumatoid arthritis can be precipitated by trauma to joints and may be associated at the time of onset with an infection that appears to be viral. The age and sex of this particular patient make a diagnosis of rheumatoid arthritis unlikely. While pleural effusions are relatively common in rheumatoid arthritis, pericardial effusions are rare. Bacterial endocarditis would be associated with all of the patient's symptoms but clear evidence of endocardial disease would be required to support such a diagnosis.

208. The answer is B. *(Hurst, ed 4. pp 306-307. Isselbacher, ed 9. p 1088.)* Normally, the second heart sound (S_2) is composed of aortic closure followed by pulmonic closure. Because inspiration increases blood return to the right side of the heart, pulmonic closure is delayed resulting in normal splitting of S_2 during inspiration. Paradoxic splitting of S_2, however, refers to a splitting of S_2 that is narrowed instead of widened with inspiration consequent to a delayed **aortic** closure. Paradoxic splitting can result from any electrical or mechanical event that delays left ventricular systole. Thus, aortic stenosis and hypertension, which increase resistance to systolic ejection of blood, delay closure of the aortic valve. Acute ischemia from angina or acute myocardial infarction also can delay ejection of blood from the left ventricle. The most common cause of paradoxic splitting—left bundle branch block—delays electrical activation of the left ventricle. Right bundle branch block results in a wide splitting of S_2 that widens further during inspiration.

209. The answer is D. *(Hurst, ed 4. pp 1004-1005. Isselbacher, ed 9. p 1099.)* The patient presented in the question has severe mitral stenosis as evidenced by her symptoms, physical examination, and calculated valve area of 0.8 cm^2 (normal range: 4 to 6 cm^2). Because of her disabling symptoms, surgery should be recommended. A loud first heart sound and an opening snap imply a noncalcified, pliable mitral valve. These findings, together with the absence of mitral regurgitation, make this patient an ideal candidate for mitral valve commissurotomy. Commissurotomy is preferred to implantation of a prosthetic valve since the former procedure carries a lower risk and avoids the long-term complications of the anticoagulation therapy that valve replacement requires. Digitalis, in the absence of rapid atrial fibrillation, would not be of significant benefit. While anticoagulant therapy is not indicated in this patient at this time, the presence of intermittent atrial fibrillation or an embolic complication would mandate the use of an anticoagulant for at least one year.

210. The answer is C. *(Hurst, ed 4. p 1208. Isselbacher, ed 9. p 1134.)* The formation of a ventricular aneurysm is a late complication of myocardial infarction and the diagnosis is usually first suggested by the presence of persistent ST-segment elevation several months after the infarction. Patients who have an aneurysm may present with arterial emboli, recurrent ventricular arrhythmias, or intractable congestive heart failure. Rupture is extremely unlikely unless there is a reinfarction over the same involved area of the ventricle. The chest x-ray occasionally reveals calcium in the wall of the aneurysm or in a mural thrombus in the middle of the aneurysm. Once confirmed by angiography, the aneurysm may be resected.

211. The answer is D. *(Isselbacher, ed 9. p 1108.)* Rheumatic heart disease still accounts for 80 percent of cases of pure or predominant aortic incompetence. The individual aortic valve cusps experience chronic inflammation, which results initially in a thickening followed by a shortening of their normal shape that prevents the formation of a tight hemodynamic seal during diastole. The chronicity of the inflammation is highlighted by the observation that there is a mean period of seven years between attacks of acute rheumatic fever and the initial experience of a hemodynamically significant episode of incompetence. It is usual for these changes in myocardial function to be asymptomatic for an even longer period, with hemodynamic disturbances being detected only by longitudinal studies of patients known to have had rheumatic fever. It may be 10 to 20 years after an attack of acute rheumatic fever before myocardial function is so compromised that symptoms result. An exaggerated awareness of the heartbeat is one of the early mild symptoms. However, symptoms may rapidly become severe; sudden death in patients with aortic incompetence is, in fact, common. Approximately 75 percent of patients with pure aortic incompetence are males, but females are more commonly found with both aortic incompetence and mitral valve disease.

212. The answer is C. *(Arnett, Curr Probl Cardiol 1:11, 14, 17-18, 1976. (Isselbacher, ed 9. pp 611, 613.)* Right-sided endocarditis has a predilection for patients who suffer from drug-abuse, alcoholism, or cancer. *Staphylococcus aureus* is the most common pathogen, followed by *Diplococcus pneumoniae.* Right-sided endocarditis often manifests as acute pneumonia. Heart murmurs in many cases are absent. In addition, the involved valve is almost always anatomically and functionally normal before the onset of the infection.

213. The answer is E. *(Isselbacher, ed 9. p 1087. Perloff, ed 2. pp 46-49, 53-54.)* Corrected transposition of the great vessels is a congenital defect involving three basic anatomic abnormalities. First, the pulmonary artery and aorta are reversed in position, the pulmonary artery lying to the right of, and inferior and posterior to, its usual site, and the aorta lying to the left of, and anterior and superior to its normal position. Second, the left-sided ventricle, which receives oxygenated blood from the lungs and left atrium, has the internal appearance of a right ventricle, and the right-sided, or venous, ventricle the appearance of a left ventricle. Third, the atrioventricular (AV) valve separating the atrium from the arterial ventricle has three cusps instead of two, and the AV valve of the venous ventricle resembles a normal mitral valve. Uncomplicated corrected transposition causes no symptoms, murmurs, or hemodynamic abnormalities since blood follows normal pathways. Corrected transposition, however, is commonly associated with (1) ventricular septal defects, (2) defects in AV conduction, and (3) abnormalities of the left AV valve. Uncomplicated transposition reveals a loud second heart sound in the second left intercostal space. Both the location and intensity of this sound, coming from aortic valve closure, may be ascribed to the anteriad and leftward position of the transposed aorta.

214. The answer is C. *(Chung, ed 2. pp 209-238. Isselbacher, ed 9. p 1057.)* The electrocardiogram presented in the question demonstrates an acute inferior wall myocardial infarction with ST-segment elevation in leads II, III, and aVF. A significant Q wave is present in lead III. The ST-segment depressions seen in the majority of the other leads are probably reciprocal changes to the ST-segment elevations mentioned. The ST-segment elevation of acute pericarditis, however, is not accompanied by reciprocal changes. Close examination of the tracing reveals P waves following each QRS complex. Whether the P wave precedes, is buried within, or follows, the QRS complex in a nodal rhythm or nodal tachycardia depends upon the location of the ectopic focus in the atrioventricular (AV) node and the rates of antegrade and retrograde conduction. In this example, the ectopic focus in the AV node reaches the ventricle just before it reaches the atrium, resulting in the P wave following the QRS complex. Nodal tachycardia is diagnosed when the rate of the pacemaker in the AV node exceeds 60 per minute. Common causes of this arrhythmia are inferior wall myocardial infarction, digitalis intoxication, and myocarditis.

215. The answer is C. *(Chung, ed 2. p 137. Isselbacher, ed 9. pp 1054-1055.)* The rhythm strip exhibited in the question reveals atrial flutter with 4:1 atrioventricular (AV) block. Atrial flutter is characterized by an atrial rate of 280 to 320 per minute; the electrocardiogram typically reveals a sawtooth baseline configuration due to the flutter waves. In the strip presented, every fourth atrial depolarization is conducted through the AV node, resulting in a ventricular rate of 75 per minute.

216. The answer is E. *(Chung, ed 2. pp 99-101. Isselbacher, ed 9. pp 1051-1052.)* The rhythm strip shown in the question reveals a blocked atrial premature contraction. The premature P wave is seen deforming the ST segment of the QRS complex that occurs prior to the pause. The atrial premature beat is blocked sinus beat. Wenckebach atrioventricular block would show gradual progression of the P-R interval prior to the blocked P wave. Similarly, sinus arrhythmia is a gradual slowing and speeding up of the heart rate; since the R-R intervals prior to the pause are perfectly equal, sinus arrhythmia is unlikely. The pause following the blocked atrial premature contraction occurs because the sinoatrial node is depolarized by the impulse, which causes it to be momentarily depressed before firing again.

217. The answer is D. *(Hurst, ed 4. pp 1266-1279. Isselbacher, ed 9. p 1135.)* The most likely diagnoses in any patient suffering acute myocardial infarction who develops severe congestive failure and a new murmur are ventricular septal defect (VSD) and papillary muscle dysfunction (PMD). While both VSD and PMD can occur with an anteroseptal infarction, VSD is the more common. The murmur of acquired VSD following infarction tends to be maximal at the lower sternal border and may be associated with a thrill. Mitral regurgitation due to PMD is usually maximal at the apex. However, it is sometimes very difficult to determine exactly which defect is present. Rupture of a papillary muscle is a catastrophic event associated with shock and intractable pulmonary edema. The hypoxemia exhibited by the patient presented in the question, while suggestive of pulmonary embolism, is compatible with severe congestive failure alone.

218. The answer is B. *(Hurst, ed 4. pp 479-501. Isselbacher, ed 9. p 1085.)* The patient discussed in the question has physical findings compatible with severe aortic stenosis. He probably has a congenital bicuspid valve that has progressively calcified. His heart signs suggest severe obstruction across the aortic valve. The fourth heart sound most likely results from contraction of the atrium against a thick, noncompliant left ventricle. Congestive failure, syncope, and chest pain indicate severe aortic stenosis; angina associated with aortic stenosis probably results from a thick ischemic, left ventricular wall. Coronary artery disease coexisting with the aortic stenosis is an additional possibility. Cardiac catheterization is indicated to define the severity of the patient's aortic stenosis. Propranolol should not be used for this patient since the decrease in contractility produced by the drug may further reduce blood flow across the aortic valve.

219. The answer is D. *(Isselbacher, ed 9. pp 1115-1116.)* In contrast to subacute bacterial endocarditis, acute bacterial endocarditis frequently develops on normal heart valves. While rheumatic and congenital malformations of the endocardium frequently act as predisposing factors for subacute bacterial endocarditis, general debilitation – especially that found in abusers of alcohol, drugs or both – is more likely to be the predisposing factor in acute endocarditis. Acute bacterial endocarditis also is a risk for older men with chronic prostatitis, particularly at the time of surgery, or for women with genitourinary infections, particularly following abortion. Although endocardial destruction may be so severe and so rapid that emergency surgery is necessary, positive blood cultures often will allow antibiotic therapy to be successfully introduced before surgery becomes necessary. In genitourinary infections, the invading organisms often are enterococci (*Streptococcus faecalis, S. faecium, S. durans*). Because these microorganisms are relatively resistant to penicillin, a combination of penicillin and gentamicin, acting synergistically against enterococci, is recommended. A daily regimen of 12 to 24 million units of penicillin G and 3 to 5 mg/kg of gentamicin usually will suffice. When acute bacterial endocarditis is caused by group D nonenterococcal organisms such as *S. bovis*, penicillin alone is quite satisfactory. An additional advantage of penicillin is the avoidance of the potential toxic effects of gentamicin. In either situation, parenteral treatment must continue for a minimum of four weeks. In patients who are allergic to penicillin, vancomycin and streptomycin are usually successful.

220. The answer is E. *(Isselbacher, ed 9. p 1247. Perloff, ed 2. pp 206-211.)* In the patient presented in the question, the absence of a history of heart murmur makes congenital heart disease an unlikely diagnosis. The rapid onset of the symptoms described makes primary pulmonary hypertension the most likely cause. While its etiology is unknown, the basic pathology of this disease involves thickening of the walls of the pulmonary arterioles resulting in progressive resistance to blood flow through the lungs. As the disease progresses, pulmonary blood flow and cardiac output are reduced and show little increase during exertion. Primary pulmonary hypertension tends to have a peak incidence in young women. Death usually occurs within four to five years after onset of symptoms. Affected patients characteristically have the symptom complex and physical findings described in the question. Systolic ejection murmurs in the pulmonic area result from ejection of blood into a proximally dilated pulmonary artery. Holosystolic murmurs at the lower left sternal border probably represent tricuspid insufficiency from right ventricular enlargement. Dilatation of the proximal portion of the pulmonary arteries, with decreased blood flow to the outer third of the lung fields, are further indications of pulmonary hypertension.

221. The answer is C. *(Isselbacher, ed 9. p 1093.)* Streptococcal antibody titers rise so consistently after streptococcal infection that they can be relied upon to help rule out respiratory tract infections caused by other organisms. Without serological evidence of a recent streptococcal infection, one should hesitate to make a diagnosis of rheumatic fever. However, two exceptions should be kept in mind. Occasionally, symptoms that are suggestive of acute rheumatic fever may not develop for as long as two months after the initial infectious episode. This is particularly the case in patients with Sydenham's chorea. As the antistreptococcal titers will have peaked before this period, the declining levels may be misleading. The situation is even more difficult in patients who have no other symptoms of rheumatic fever besides a pancarditis. In such cases, it may be several months after the acute infection before a diagnosis is made. Such patients may have low antibody titers when seen initially.

222. The answer is D. *(Hurst, ed 4. pp 1571-1572. Isselbacher, ed 9. p 1142.)* Long-term alcohol abuse has a direct toxic effect on the myocardium. The patient who has alcoholic cardiomyopathy may present with dyspnea on exertion or with palpitations. Unexplained sinus tachycardia, premature ventricular contractions, or atrial fibrillation may be present. With continued alcohol abuse, overt left and right ventricular failure develop. Alcohol increases cardiac output in normal individuals by increasing the heart rate. In addition to standard modes of therapy for congestive failure, complete abstinence from alcohol is necessary to prevent further decompensation and, in some patients, to allow for recovery.

223. The answer is A. *(Forrester, N Engl J Med 205:1356-1360, 1976. Isselbacher, ed 9. p 1277.)* The Swan-Ganz pulmonary artery catheter provides an accurate bedside means of determining left ventricular filling pressures. The catheter is passed through a vein to the heart where it is placed in a pulmonary artery. When the balloon at the tip is inflated, the catheter records pulmonary capillary pressure, which is equivalent to left atrial pressure and, in the absence of mitral stenosis, to left ventricular diastolic pressure. The level of pulmonary capillary pressure correlates with left ventricular volume. Normal pulmonary capillary pressure is 5 to 12 mm Hg. Levels above 18 to 20 mm Hg are associated with signs of congestive heart failure. On admission to the hospital, the patient presented in the question had bibasilar rales, which probably resulted from his cigarette smoking, since an S_3 gallop, which would have suggested congestive failure, was not heard. His postdiuretic pulmonary capillary pressure of 4 mm Hg is low and indicates hypovolemia. Appropriate therapy for this patient would be to administer intravenous fluids to bring his pulmonary capillary pressure up to at least 10 to 12 mm Hg.

224. The answer is B. *(Isselbacher, ed 9. p 1125.)* Exercise testing under carefully controlled conditions can safely place a hemodynamic load on the myocardium that, in the presence of ischemic disease, will produce characteristic electrocardiographic changes. Because of the ability of stress testing to provide early warning of potential ischemic episodes in asymptomatic patients, its use in routine physical examinations, particularly in men over the age of 35, is rapidly increasing. Longitudinal studies of young personnel in the armed forces who had an abnormal exercise tolerance test, in spite of an absence of symptoms, have revealed that this group indeed is at risk for developing angina, myocardial infarction, and even sudden death. A diagnosis of ischemic heart disease by stress testing often can be followed by preventive measures that will delay or minimize subsequent clinical episodes of ischemic heart disease. The role of arteriography and corrective bypass surgery in such patients remains controversial and will not be settled until more data are available from longitudinal studies. In determining whether angiography is needed in a particular case, the following factors should be considered: (1) Were the abnormalities noted extreme? For example, a 4 mm ST-segment depression occurring after a short period of mild exercise; (2) In which electrocardiographic leads did the changes predominate? For example, changes in anterior leads have a worse prognosis than those in inferior leads; (3) The patient's age; (4) The patient's occupation. The pilot described in the question clearly should have angiography; a 75-year-old man, all things considered, probably should not.

225. The answer is A. *(Bellet, pp 138-139. Isselbacher, ed 9. pp 1061-1062.)* The first part of the rhythm strip shown in the question demonstrates Mobitz II atrioventricular (AV) block with every other P wave conducted to the ventricles. A ventricular premature contraction is then noted, followed by P waves without any QRS complexes. There is complete lack of conduction of the atrial impulses and, furthermore, a lack of any subsidiary pacemaker to maintain cardiac rhythm. The most appropriate immediate therapy for this conduction problem would be cardiopulmonary resuscitation and infusion of isoproterenol. Isoproterenol increases automaticity of cardiac pacemakers and thus may provoke a subsidiary pacemaker to start firing. Atropine might be useful except that the presence of Mobitz II block and wide QRS complexes suggests disease below the AV node, where atropine exerts little effect on subsidiary pacemakers. Intracardiac epinephrine should be used only as a last resort.

226. The answer is B. *(Chung, ed 2. pp 593-595. Isselbacher, ed 9. p 1047.)* The rhythm strip displayed in the question reveals paced rhythm with 100 percent capture at a rate of 60 per minute. P waves can be seen marching through, independent of the QRS complexes, at a rate of 65 per minute. The diagnosis in this case is made by the finding of pacing spikes preceding each QRS complex. In this case, although the atria are firing at 65 beats per minute, the impulses are being blocked, which results in a slow ventricular rate and the need for a pacemaker.

227. The answer is E. *(Chung, ed 2. p 314. Isselbacher, ed 9. p 1059.)* The rhythm strip exhibited both in the question and below reveals a P wave before the first QRS complex, with a short P-R interval. The P waves then move into the QRS complexes until the end of the strip where a P wave is again seen preceding a QRS complex. The P-P intervals and the QRS intervals are almost identical. This strip reveals atrioventricular (AV) dissociation in which the atria are being depolarized by the sinus node and the ventricles are being depolarized by a junctional or AV nodal focus. This particular example of AV dissociation is termed "isorhythmic dissociation" since the rates of atria and ventricles are almost equal. The preferred meaning of AV dissociation implies two separate pacemakers, with the lower focus faster in rate than the higher focus. This situation differs from complete heart block, in which the rate of the lower focus is slower than the higher, since it is an escape rhythm. In AV dissociation, the lower focus is firing faster than the higher because of increased automaticity and thus controlling the ventricles only because it is firing faster than the sinus node. AV dissociation is commonly associated with digitalis toxicity, inferior wall myocardial infarction, and hypokalemia.

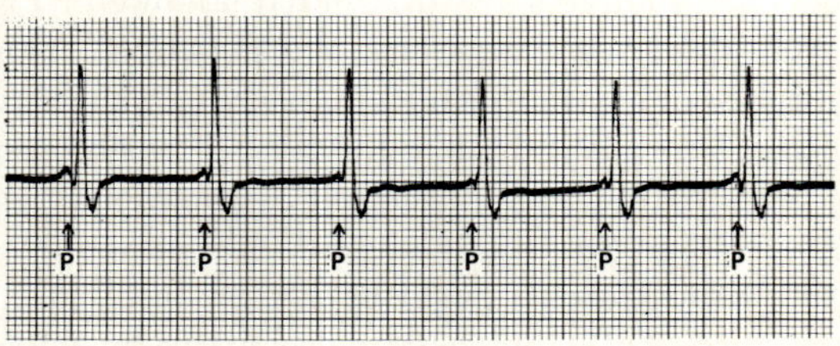

228-231. The answers are: 228-E, 229-D, 230-B, 231-A. *(Hurst, ed 4. pp 309-310. Isselbacher, ed 9. p 1010.)* Hyperkalemia decreases the rate of spontaneous diastolic depolarization in all pacemaker cells. It also results in slowing of conduction. One of the earliest electrocardiographic signs of hyperkalemia is the appearance of tall, peaked T waves. More severe elevations of the serum potassium result in widening of the QRS complex.

Hypokalemia typically increases automaticity of myocardial fibers, resulting in ectopic beats or arrhythmias. Electrocardiography in hypokalemia reveals flattening of the T wave and prominent U waves.

Hypocalcemia results in prolongation of the Q-T interval, most commonly when the serum calcium level falls below 6 mg/100 ml. Low serum calcium levels tend to decrease myocardial contractility.

At serum sodium levels compatible with life, neither hyponatremia nor hypernatremia results in any characteristic electrocardiographic abnormalities.

232-235. The answers are: 232-D, 233-A, 234-B, 235-D. *(Hurst, ed 4. pp 596-597. Isselbacher, ed 9. p 1059. Mason, pp 333, 338-339.)* Patients with chronic obstructive lung disease tolerate digitalis less well than the general population. This is thought to result from the effect that hypoxemia has on the binding of digitalis to ATPase localized on cell membranes. All forms of digitalis toxicity occur more frequently in this population than in patients who do not have obstructive lung disease, therefore appropriate attention to dosage administration schedules is warranted.

Patients with severe pericardial effusion depend on high filling pressures in the cardiac chambers to maintain cardiac output in the face of an effusion that tends to limit both filling and emptying of the heart. Diuretics may reduce this filling pressure and produce cardiac failure.

Digitalis has side effects that cause cardiac problems, but it also has a number of extra-cardiac side effects including gynecomastia, the development of yellowish-green sputum, and severe headaches.

In patients with ventricular tachycardia who are receiving large doses of quinidine, the cardiac rhythm may fail to revert to sinus rhythm after cardioversion. The ventricular rate may slow to 120 beats per minute or less. Under these circumstances, the administration of atropine (up to 2 mg intravenously) may increase the atrial rate to a level that exceeds the ventricular rate and allows recapture of the conducting system by the sinoatrial node.

236-239. The answers are: 236-B, 237-E, 238-D, 239-A. *(Hurst, ed 4. pp 1448-1451. Isselbacher, ed 9. pp 391, 393-394, 1043.)* Hydralazine's mode of action as an antihypertensive agent is by a direct vasodilating action on peripheral vessels. Because the drug tends to cause an increase in heart rate, it must be used cautiously in the patient who has angina.

Clonidine is a newly developed agent that inhibits central nervous system sympathetic discharge, which in turn results in a decrease in peripheral resistance.

Guanethidine works peripherally on the nerve terminals. This agent interferes with the release of norepinephrine, at the same time depleting the nerve endings of norepinephrine.

Propranolol is a beta-blocking agent that has several possible mechanisms of action in hypertension. In some patients, the drug may lower blood pressure by a reduction in cardiac output. The predominant action apparently derives from propranolol's ability to decrease renin release, a rationale that is supported by the finding that this drug is most effective in cases of "high renin" hypertension.

240-242. The answers are: 240-A, 241-D, 242-C. *(Isselbacher, ed 9. pp 463, 1076, 1426, 2012.)* Dextrocardia is a prominent feature of Kartagener's syndrome, an inherited condition that features situs inversus, chronic sinusitis, and bronchiectasis.

Aortic and pulmonary artery dilatation commonly occur with the inborn error of metabolism, homocystinuria. This condition, which is caused by a deficiency of the enzyme cystathionine synthetase, is characterized by the presence of intravascular thrombosis, lens subluxation, and osteoporosis, as well as large vessel dilatation.

Hyperextensible joints, one of the common defects in Down's syndrome (trisomy 21), is frequently associated with cardiac abnormalities, including an endocardial cushion defect, atrial and ventrical septal defects, and the tetralogy of Fallot. Hypotonia often accompanies the hyperextensible joints. Mongoloid facies and mental retardation are regularly associated with this syndrome.

243-247. The answers are: 243-A, 244-D, 245-E, 246-B, 247-A. *(Hurst, ed 4. pp 75-76, 571-572. Isselbacher, ed 9. pp 994-995.)* The normal jugular venous pulse wave consists of three positive waves and two troughs. Normally, the *a* wave is the largest wave and is due to right atrial contraction. The *c* wave that follows is probably related to bulging of the tricuspid valve into the atrium. Relaxation of the atrium results in the *x* descent. The *v* wave results from filling of the right atrium with blood while the tricuspid valve is still closed. The *y* descent is the result of opening of the tricuspid valve. An S_4 gallop is produced by atrial contraction and thus would occur at approximately the same time as the *a* wave.

Thus, abnormally large *a* waves would be expected in situations in which the right atrium is contracting against increased resistance such as with tricuspid stenosis, pulmonic stenosis, or pulmonary hypertension. Moderate or severe tricuspid regurgitation typically causes obliteration of the normal *x* descent. When

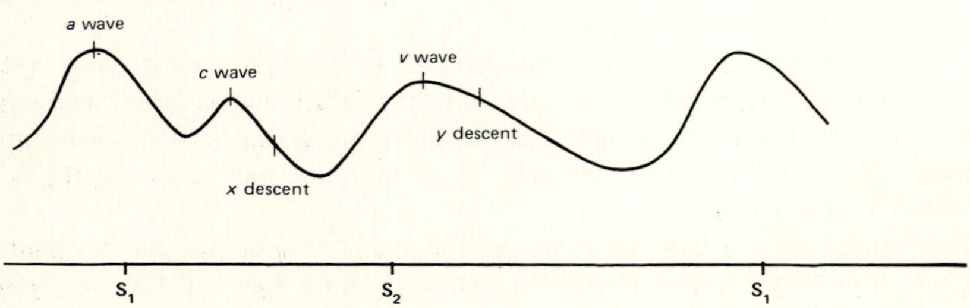

regurgitation is severe, the *c* and *v* waves may merge, resulting in a single, large *v* wave. Obstruction to right atrial emptying would be expected to result in a slow *y* descent, which is classically seen with tricuspid stenosis. A prominent *y* descent is characteristic of constrictive pericarditis.

248-250. The answers are: 248-D, 249-B, 250-C. *(Hurst, ed 4. pp 282, 402-403, 777.)* Ebstein's anomaly of the tricuspid valve consists of an abnormality in which the leaflets of the tricuspid valve arise from the wall of the right ventricle rather than the valve ring. In addition, the upper portion of the right ventricle is abnormally thin and continuous with the right atrium. Tricuspid regurgitation is commonly present.

An anomalous coronary artery arising from the pulmonary artery produces essentially a left-to-right shunt; blood from a normal coronary artery passes through collateral vessels to this anomalous artery and thus is diverted into the pulmonary circulation. As the affected patient enters adolescence, myocardial blood supply becomes inadequate and cardiomegaly, congestive failure, mitral regurgitation, or myocardial infarction results.

Ostium secundum atrial septal defect is the common form of interatrial communication. Blood flows from the left atrium through the defect into the right heart. The increased flow across the right ventricular outflow tract creates a "relative" pulmonic stenosis with a systolic ejection murmur heard in the second left intercostal space; the murmur does not result from flow across the atrial septal defect. In addition, there is a widely split second heart sound that is not affected by respiration.

251-253. The answers are: 251-D, 252-B, 253-A. *(Hurst, ed 4. pp 199, 1049, 1056. Isselbacher, ed 9. pp 1107, 1110, 1154.)* Tricuspid stenosis is characterized by a slow *y* descent of the jugular pulse and a diastolic rumble at the lower left sternal border.

Aortic regurgitation, in addition to generating the characteristic decrescendo diastolic murmur along the left sternal border, may also cause a diastolic rumble at the apex. Termed an Austin Flint murmur, this diastolic rumble is thought to result from the regurgitant jet of blood hitting the anterior leaflet of the mitral valve. Although distinguishing this murmur from that of mitral stenosis may be difficult, the absence of both an opening snap and loud first heart sound should suggest an Austin Flint murmur.

Constrictive pericarditis is characterized by a sharp *y* descent; this diagnosis should be considered in any patient who has unexplained edema or ascites.

Endocrinology and Metabolic Disease

DIRECTIONS: Each question below contains five suggested answers. Choose the **one best** response to each question.

254. A 25-year-old woman who has insulin-dependent diabetes develops recurrent hypoglycemia. Her history reveals amenorrhea of two months duration. A urinalysis is negative for glucose and protein; a vaginal smear shows no evidence of estrogen deficiency. The most likely diagnosis is

(A) pregnancy
(B) renal failure
(C) hypopituitarism
(D) insulinoma
(E) hyperthyroidism

255. Diabetic neuropathy may cause all the following clinical conditions EXCEPT

(A) plantar ulcer
(B) necrobiosis lipoidica diabeticorum
(C) Charcot's joints
(D) orthostatic hypotension
(E) impotence

256. An otherwise healthy 60-year-old man is noted on routine examination to have a firm thyroid nodule. Serum thyroxine is 8.0 μg/100 ml (normal: 4 to 11). Thyroid scan demonstrates a "cold" nodule, and ultrasonography reveals that the mass is solid. The most appropriate management would be which of the following procedures?

(A) Complete lobectomy
(B) Needle biopsy
(C) Exogenous thyroid suppression
(D) Radioactive iodine therapy
(E) External irradiation

257. A patient develops severe hypotension immediately after removal of a pheochromocytoma. The most appropriate management would be the administration of which of the following?

(A) Corticosteroids
(B) Mineralocorticoids
(C) Alpha-stimulating agents
(D) Beta-stimulating agents
(E) Blood or plasma

258. A 38-year-old man, who has noted over the past year a steady decline in his ability to achieve an erection, now is unable to achieve one under any circumstances. He continues to need to shave, although less frequently than before. Physical examination reveals masculine features, normal testes, and a normal penis. Plasma testosterone is 0.03 μg/100 ml (normal: 0.3 to 1.0). Serum gonadotropins and urinary 17-ketosteroids are normal. The next step in the management of this patient would be to

(A) obtain a psychiatric evaluation
(B) perform a glucose tolerance test
(C) evaluate pituitary function
(D) administer testosterone
(E) perform a testicular biopsy

259. A patient who has a history of hypercalcemia, hypophosphatemia, and recurrent renal stones is diagnosed as having primary hyperparathyroidism on the basis of elevated parathormone levels and increased cyclic AMP excretion. Neck exploration has failed to locate the adenoma. The most useful procedure for localizing the tumor in this patient would be which of the following?

(A) Barium swallow
(B) Venous parathormone determination
(C) Selenium methionine scan
(D) Arteriography
(E) Retrograde venography

260. A 45-year-old diabetic man, found lying on the floor and unresponsive, is admitted to a hospital. He has been treated with 30 units of NPH insulin daily for the past six years. His fasting blood glucose level was 125 mg/100 ml two months before admission. Two weeks prior to admission, the patient developed angina and was given propranolol. Physical examination shows a blood pressure of 110/60 mm Hg, pulse 90/minute and regular, spontaneous respirations, and temperature of 35.5°C (95.9°F). He is responsive only to pain. Blood serum drawn on admission is turbid. The physician should immediately take which of the following steps?

(A) Perform a lumbar puncture
(B) Start intravenous 5% dextrose
(C) Give intravenous glucose, 25 g
(D) Obtain an electrocardiogram
(E) Call the laboratory for results of blood tests

261. Nonketotic hyperosmolar coma generally occurs in the maturity-onset diabetic patient, and in middle-aged or elderly subjects without a history of diabetes. This syndrome may be precipitated by all the following EXCEPT

(A) thiazide diuretics
(B) phenformin (DBI)
(C) phenytoin (Dilantin)
(D) peritoneal dialysis
(E) extensive burns

262. A 42-year-old woman is evaluated for hypoglycemia. She has experienced recurrent episodes of inappropriate behavior and dizziness for the past year, and she had syncope on one occasion after mowing her lawn. She denies hunger or palpitations and only occasionally has noted sweating. The patient has gained 15 pounds during the past year. Laboratory plasma studies reveal a glucose level of 65 mg/100 ml, insulin level of 18 μU/ml (normal: 10 to 20) after an overnight fast, and a diabetic glucose tolerance test (two hour value: 225 mg/100 ml) without reactive hypoglycemia. After 48 hours of fasting, the patient became confused. At this time her plasma glucose and insulin levels are 34 mg/100 ml and 20 μU/ml, respectively. The most likely diagnosis is

(A) Addison's disease
(B) reactive hypoglycemia
(C) diabetes mellitus
(D) insulinoma
(E) hepatoma

263. A 6-year-old girl develops breast tissue, pubic hair, and begins menstruating. The most likely diagnosis is which of the following?

(A) Constitutional sexual precocity
(B) Ovarian tumor
(C) Adrenal tumor
(D) McCune-Albright syndrome
(E) Pinealoma

264. A 60-year-old woman who has been aware of a swelling in her neck for many years presents with generalized muscle weakness, loss of appetite, and palpitations. An electrocardiogram reveals rapid atrial fibrillation. Despite adequate digitalization, there is little slowing of her ventricular rate. Thyroid function studies reveal a serum thyroxine level of 12 μg/100 ml (normal: 5 to 12), with a triiodothyronine (T_3) level of 200 ng/100 ml (normal: 80 to 160), as measured by radioimmunoassay. In respect to this patient's disorder, the most appropriate diagnosis and treatment would be

(A) typical Graves' disease; therapy with antithyroid drugs
(B) toxic multinodular goiter; therapy with antithyroid drugs followed by surgery
(C) toxic multinodular goiter; initiation of therapy with 10 μCi/g of ^{131}I
(D) toxic multinodular goiter; initiation of therapy with antithyroid agents followed by 20 μCi/g of ^{131}I when euthyroid
(E) toxic multinodular goiter; initiation of therapy with propranolol and antithyroid agents followed by 20 μCi of ^{131}I when euthyroid

265. An active 24-year-old woman is found to have Hodgkin's disease on the basis of a cervical node biopsy. Chest x-ray reveals an anterior mediastinal mass, but lymphangiogram and liver biopsy are negative. Radiotherapy to the involved lymph nodes results in clinical remission; however, two months later the patient develops clinical and laboratory evidence of hypothyroidism. The most likely cause for hypothyroidism in this patient is

(A) Hashimoto's thyroiditis
(B) iodine deficiency
(C) iodine excess
(D) lymphomatous infiltration of the thyroid
(E) hypopituitarism

266. A 30-year-old man is evaluated for a thyroid nodule. The patient reports that his father died from "thyroid cancer" and that a brother had a history of recurrent renal stones. Blood calcitonin concentration is 2000 pg/ml (normal: less than 100); serum calcium and phosphate levels are normal. Before referring the patient to a surgeon, the physician should

(A) obtain a liver scan
(B) perform a calcium infusion test
(C) measure urinary catecholamines
(D) administer suppressive doses of thyroxine and measure levels of thyroid stimulating hormone
(E) treat the patient with radioactive iodine

267. A 55-year-old woman who has a history of severe depression and who had radical mastectomy for carcinoma of the breast one year previously, develops polyuria, nocturia, and excessive thirst. Laboratory values are:

Serum electrolytes (mEq/L): Na^+ 149; K^+ 3.6
Serum calcium: 9.5 mg/100 ml
Blood glucose: 110 mg/100 ml
Blood urea nitrogen: 30 mg/100 ml
Urine osmolality 150 mOsm/kg

The most likely diagnosis is

(A) psychogenic polydipsia
(B) renal glycosuria
(C) hypercalciuria
(D) diabetes insipidus
(E) inappropriate antidiuretic hormone syndrome

268. A 32-year-old woman has a three-year history of oligomenorrhea that has progressed to amenorrhea during the past year. She has observed loss of breast fullness, reduced hip measurements, acne, increased body hair, and deepening of her voice. Physical examination reveals frontal balding, clitoral hypertrophy, and a male escutcheon. Urinary 17-hydroxycorticoid and 17-ketosteroid levels are normal. Plasma testosterone level is 6 ng/ml (normal: 0.2 to 0.8). The most likely diagnosis of this patient's disorder is

(A) hilar cell tumor
(B) Cushing's syndrome
(C) arrhenoblastoma
(D) polycystic ovary syndrome
(E) granulosa-theca cell tumor

269. A 25-year-old woman who is slender and slow of speech complains of fatigue and anorexia. Physical examination reveals a blood pressure of 110/80 mm Hg supine and 80/60 mm Hg standing, pigment in the palmar creases and on the buccal mucosa, and several discrete areas of depigmentation on the neck and shoulders. Pubic and axillary hair is sparse; the thyroid is twice normal size; deep tendon reflexes are mildly depressed. Laboratory values are:

Serum electrolytes (mEq/L): Na^+ 110; K^+ 6.2; Cl^- 70; HCO_3^- 18
Blood glucose: 190 mg/100 ml
Blood urea nitrogen: 30 mg/100 ml
Thyroid antibodies: positive

The most likely diagnosis in this patient is

(A) hypothyroidism
(B) Addison's disease
(C) Schmidt's syndrome
(D) pituitary adenoma
(E) inappropriate antidiuretic hormone

270. A 35-year-old woman has a six-month history of amenorrhea. A five-day course of medroxyprogesterone acetate (Provera), 10 mg, fails to induce withdrawal bleeding, while vaginal bleeding occurs following twenty days of conjugated estrogen (1.25 mg) administration. Her serum luteinizing and follicle-stimulating hormones are markedly increased. These findings are most consistent with which of the following abnormalities?

(A) Pituitary adenoma
(B) Polycystic ovary syndrome
(C) Endometrial failure
(D) Premature menopause
(E) Psychiatric illness

271. The most satisfactory daily replacement therapy for a patient with complete adrenal failure is

(A) prednisone, 15 mg in the morning and late afternoon
(B) cortisone acetate, 25 mg in the morning, 12.5 mg in the late afternoon
(C) cortisone acetate, 25 mg in the morning, 50 mg in the late afternoon
(D) cortisone acetate, 25 mg in the morning, 12.5 mg in the late afternoon with 0.1 mg 9α-fluorohydrocortisone
(E) cortisone acetate, 25 mg in the morning, 50 mg in the late afternoon with 0.2 mg 9α-fluorohydrocortisone

272. A 43-year-old man presents with a headache, muscle weakness, and fatigue. His blood pressure is 150/120 mm Hg; he has mild congestive heart failure. An electrocardiogram shows prominent U waves and premature ventricular contractions, together with evidence of left ventricular enlargement. He is given furosemide 40 mg daily, and returns for evaluation two months later. His serum level of sodium is then 145 mEq/L, potassium 2.8 mEq/L, bicarbonate 30 mEq/L. The next step in the management of this patient should be to

(A) estimate plasma renin activity
(B) estimate plasma renin activity during volume depletion
(C) measure plasma aldosterone following intravenous saline loading
(D) discontinue furosemide therapy
(E) discontinue furosemide therapy and administer potassium chloride supplements

273. The antiserotonergic agent, cyproheptadine, has been used with initial success in the treatment of

(A) acromegaly
(B) Cushing's syndrome
(C) the Stein-Leventhal syndrome
(D) the galactorrhea-amenorrhea syndrome
(E) none of the above

274. A 27-year-old woman presents with shortness of breath. Her radiological skeletal survey is negative. Laboratory serum values are as follows:

Chloride: 98 mEq/L
Calcium: 11.9 mg/100 ml (nl 9-11)
Phosphorus: 3.6 mg/100 ml (nl 3-4.5)
Uric acid: 8.5 mg/100 ml (nl 2.5-5.5)
Alkaline phosphatase: 50 U/L (nl 21-91)

Blood urea nitrogen is 20 mg/100 ml. Pulmonary function tests reveal reduced vital capacity and reduced carbon monoxide diffusing capacity. Flat plate x-ray of the abdomen reveals bilateral nephrocalcinosis. The appropriate treatment for this patient is

(A) parathyroid exploration followed by subtotal parathyroidectomy
(B) potassium phosphate, 2 g daily
(C) mithramycin, 25 μg/kg body weight
(D) furosemide, 40 mg daily
(E) prednisone, 15 mg daily

275. The patient pictured below complains of the sudden onset of a painful "lump" in her neck following an upper respiratory infection. Physical examination reveals a soft, round, tender, midline mass at the level of the hyoid bone. The most likely diagnosis is

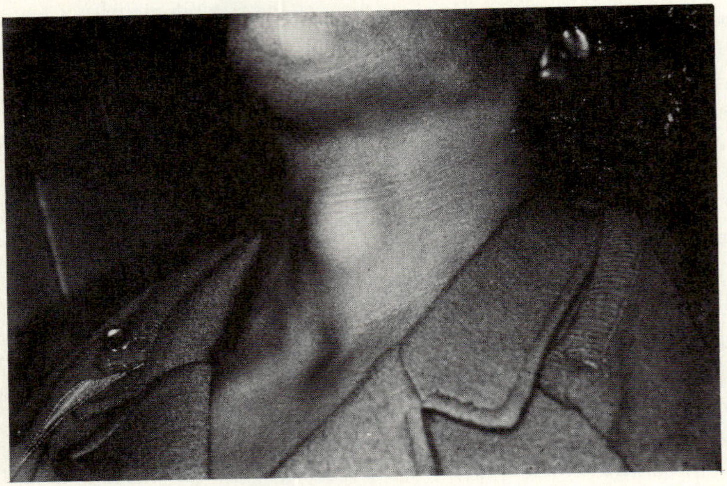

(A) acute suppurative thyroiditis
(B) subacute thyroiditis
(C) thyroglossal duct cyst
(D) toxic nodular goiter
(E) thyroid adenoma

DIRECTIONS: Each question below contains four suggested answers of which **one** or **more** is correct. Choose the answer:

A	if	**1, 2, and 3**	are correct
B	if	**1 and 3**	are correct
C	if	**2 and 4**	are correct
D	if	**4**	is correct
E	if	**1, 2, 3, and 4**	are correct

276. A 20-year-old man who has a history of polyuria and hypotonic urine is placed on restricted water intake. After a period of dehydration, his urine osmolality stabilizes at 450 mOsm/kg. Following injection of vasopressin (Pitressin) his urine osmolality rises to 600 mOsm/kg. This patient's symptoms are likely to improve if he is treated with

(1) oral chlorpropamide
(2) thiazide diuretics
(3) lysine-vasopressin nasal spray
(4) oral tolbutamide

277. Hyperparathyroidism may be associated with which of the following abnormalities?

(1) Moniliasis
(2) Personality disturbances
(3) Prolonged Q-T interval on electrocardiogram
(4) Intense pruritus

278. Addisonian crisis is characterized by which of the following clinical findings?

(1) Diarrhea
(2) Hypotension
(3) Nausea and vomiting
(4) Hypothermia

279. Concurrent hypocalcemia and hyperphosphatemia is associated with

(1) malabsorption
(2) rickets
(3) pancreatitis
(4) renal failure

280. Patients afflicted with active Paget's disease (ostetitis deformans) generally demonstrate elevated levels of which of the following substances?

(1) Serum alkaline phosphatase
(2) Serum calcium
(3) Urine hydroxyproline
(4) Urine calcium

281. Correct statements concerning hyperosmolar nonketotic diabetic coma include which of the following?

(1) It is usually a complication of juvenile-onset diabetes
(2) The mortality rate in hyperosmolar coma is significantly higher than in diabetic ketoacidosis
(3) Potassium salts are usually required later in the treatment of hyperosmolar coma than in ketoacidosis because of the absence of acidosis
(4) Ketone concentrations of 4-6 mOsm/kg are frequent

SUMMARY OF DIRECTIONS

A	B	C	D	E
1, 2, 3 only	1, 3 only	2, 4 only	4 only	All are correct

282. Cushing's syndrome is characterized by which of the following statements?

(1) Circulating eosinophils are below 100 cells/mm^3 in 90 percent of cases
(2) Although truncal obesity is generally present, a redistribution of weight is characteristic and approximately half the affected patients exhibit no weight gain
(3) Adrenal hyperplasia secondary to either pituitary or nonendocrine ACTH production can often be distinguished by a high-dosage dexamethasone suppression test
(4) The dexamethasone suppression test is less useful in screening for this syndrome than the now generally available radioimmunoassay for ACTH

283. A 25-year-old woman complains of a recent onset of nervousness, palpitations, and increased sweating. Her serum thyroxine is 15 μg/100 ml (normal: 4 to 11), and radioactive iodine uptake is 1 percent. Hyperthyroidism in this patient may have been induced by

(1) exogenous thyroid
(2) pituitary adenoma
(3) cholecystography
(4) oat cell carcinoma of the lungs

284. Hypercalcemia in sarcoidosis is associated with

(1) seasonal changes in serum calcium
(2) improvement following corticosteroid therapy
(3) reduced parathormone concentration
(4) brown tumors

285. X-ray findings associated with hyperparathyroidism include

(1) subperiosteal resorption of the phalanges
(2) pseudofractures
(3) dissolution of phalangeal tufts
(4) osteosclerosis

286. Correct statements concerning diabetic retinopathy include which of the following?

(1) Cotton wool exudates are caused by microinfarcts
(2) Hard exudates reflect old, healed microinfarcts
(3) A sudden increase in the number of cotton wool exudates is a serious prognostic sign
(4) Cotton wool exudates are much more common than hard exudates

287. Osteoporosis may be distinguished from osteomalacia on the basis of

(1) serum calcium
(2) pseudofractures
(3) serum alkaline phosphatase
(4) urinary calcium

288. Klinefelter's syndrome may be associated with which of the following endocrinologic manifestations?

(1) Gynecomastia
(2) High follicle-stimulating hormone levels
(3) Infertility
(4) Normal testosterone levels

289. Correct statements about Kallmann's syndrome (hypogonadotropic hypogonadism) include which of the following?

(1) Affected patients usually have small, hard testes
(2) It is associated with anosmia
(3) Affected patients are usually short
(4) Luteinizing hormone (LH) secretion can be stimulated in affected patients by LH-releasing factor

290. Hyperaldosteronism is often associated with

(1) diuretic therapy
(2) Cushing's syndrome
(3) malignant hypertension
(4) licorice ingestion

291. Gynecomastia may be associated with which of the following situations?

(1) Cirrhosis
(2) Digitalis administration
(3) Puberty
(4) Hyperthyroidism

292. Toxic nodular goiter (Plummer's disease) may be associated with

(1) exophthalmos
(2) thyroid acropathy
(3) pretibial myxedema
(4) onycholysis

293. Propylthiouracil inhibits which of the following thyroid processes?

(1) Thyroid release
(2) Conversion of T_4 to T_3
(3) Active iodine transport
(4) Organification

294. Correct statements concerning diabetes insipidus include which of the following?

(1) A dehydration test requires withholding fluids until there is a loss in body weight of at least 4 kg
(2) A new synthetic analog of vasopressin, desmopressin acetate (DDAVP), is more effective than synthetic lypressin (DIAPID) in that its effect lasts from 12 to 24 hours
(3) Ethacrynic acid provides effective therapy
(4) Water intoxication with normal diluting capacity has been reported in patients given thioridazine (Mellaril)

295. A 30-year-old man complains of headaches. A skull x-ray shows enlargement of the sella turcica. These findings are consistent with a diagnosis of

(1) pituitary adenoma
(2) craniopharyngioma
(3) empty-sella syndrome
(4) internal carotid artery aneurysm

SUMMARY OF DIRECTIONS

A	B	C	D	E
1, 2, 3 only	1, 3 only	2, 4 only	4 only	All are correct

296. A patient who has undergone bilateral adrenalectomy for Cushing's syndrome develops a deep tan in winter. In evaluating this patient, the physician should consider the possibility of

(1) residual ectopic adrenal tissue
(2) a pituitary tumor
(3) iatrogenic Cushing's syndrome
(4) inadequate adrenal replacement

297. Hyperprolactinemia is characterized by which of the following observations?

(1) It may occur in the absence of galactorrhea
(2) It may be reduced by L-dopa in the presence of a pituitary tumor
(3) It may be caused by phenothiazines
(4) It may cause gynecomastia

298. A 15-year-old boy, hospitalized for a fractured pelvis, is restricted to complete bedrest. Which of the following laboratory abnormalities may result?

(1) Glucose intolerance
(2) Hypercalcemia
(3) Absent diurnal steroid rhythm
(4) Hyperparathyroidism

299. Correct statements regarding the laboratory findings in patients who have Cushing's syndrome include which of the following?

(1) The presence of an abnormal diurnal steroid rhythm is diagnostic of the disorder
(2) An abnormal overnight dexamethasone suppression test (1 mg) is diagnostic of the disorder
(3) An exaggerated increase in plasma cortisol is usually observed following insulin-induced hypoglycemia
(4) Normal urinary 17-hydroxycorticosteroids are observed in 10 to 15 percent of affected patients

300. Recent studies on diabetic ketoacidosis have revealed that

(1) ketone production is associated with increased activity of carnitine acyltransferase
(2) hypophosphatemia usually becomes manifest within 4-12 hours of institution of therapy
(3) an advantage of low-dose insulin therapy is the diminished incidence of hypoglycemia and hypokalemia
(4) a nitroprusside reaction, which is a qualitative test for ketone, may be negative because of a high acetoacetate/β-hydroxybutyrate ratio

301. Correct statements about thyroid antibodies include which of the following?

(1) They may be observed in elderly women
(2) They may be observed in pernicious anemia
(3) They are usually observed in Hashimoto's thyroiditis
(4) They are usually observed in subacute thyroiditis

302. Correct statements concerning subacute thyroiditis (de Quervain's thyroiditis) include which of the following?

(1) Pain, both localized and referred, is characteristic
(2) The erythrocyte sedimentation rate is increased and radioactive iodine uptake decreased
(3) The thyroid is extremely tender and occasionally nodular
(4) An elevated protein-bound iodine level is commonly found

303. Diabetic retinopathy is characterized by which of the following statements?

(1) It usually can be treated with improved glucose regulation
(2) Blindness may result in the absence of proliferative changes
(3) Once established, it is invariably progressive
(4) It is present in 50 percent of patients who have had diabetes for ten years

304. A thin, 30-year-old woman complains of nervousness, mild sweating, palpitations, scanty menses, and weight loss. Her blood pressure is 150/80 mm Hg and pulse rate 96/minute. She displays mild hyperpigmentation and telangiectasia on the face. A small thyroid nodule is palpable. Serum thyroxine is 9.0 μg/100 ml (normal: 4.5 to 10); resin T_3 uptake is normal; radioactive iodine uptake is 30 percent (normal: 5 to 35); and thyroid scan shows uptake by a solitary left-sided thyroid nodule (no uptake by the right lobe). The diagnosis of hyperthyroidism in this patient may be established by

(1) T_3 suppression test
(2) serum long-acting thyroid stimulator assay
(3) serum triiodothyronine radioimmunoassay
(4) serum thyroid-stimulating hormone assay

305. After an initial two to three hours of insulin treatment for diabetic ketoacidosis, there is most often a significant decline in blood level of

(1) glucose
(2) β-hydroxybutyrate
(3) free fatty acids
(4) acetoacetate

306. Bromocriptine is recently reported to have been successful in the treatment of

(1) male infertility associated with hyperprolactinemia
(2) female infertility associated with hyperprolactinemia
(3) acromegaly
(4) the Chiari-Frommel syndrome

SUMMARY OF DIRECTIONS

A	B	C	D	E
1, 2, 3 only	1, 3 only	2, 4 only	4 only	All are correct

307. In a controlled study of oral hypoglycemic agents, the University Group Diabetes Program concluded that

(1) tolbutamide (Orinase) increases the risk of death from cardiovascular causes
(2) overall mortality rates are not statistically different between tolbutamide and diet-treated groups
(3) phenformin increases the risk of death from cardiovascular causes
(4) insulin decreases the risk of death from cardiovascular causes

308. An elderly man, found to be unresponsive, is brought to the emergency room. Although he is a victim of chronic alcoholism, his breath does not smell of alcohol. The patient apparently had been drinking the previous day, but friends claim that he did not drink on the day he was brought to the hospital. His appetite had been poor during the past week. Laboratory values are:

Serum electrolytes (mEq/L): Na^+ 142; Cl^- 95; HCO_3^- 15
Serum ketones: large, undiluted
Blood glucose: 30 mg/100 ml
Blood urea nitrogen: 8 mg/100 ml
Blood alcohol: 10 mg/100 ml (intoxication: over 100 mg/100 ml)

The findings in this patient justify which of the following statements?

(1) After the patient has completely recovered, a trial of alcohol ingestion would be expected to produce hypoglycemia
(2) The presence of hyperketonemia rules out hyperinsulinism as a cause of hypoglycemia
(3) The relatively low blood alcohol levels make the diagnosis of alcohol-induced hypoglycemia unlikely
(4) Normal or only mildly abnormal liver function test results would be expected in this patient

DIRECTIONS: The groups of questions below consist of lettered choices followed by several numbered items. For each numbered item select the **one** lettered choice with which it is **most** closely associated. Each lettered choice may be used once, more than once, or not at all.

Questions 309-312

For each case presentation that follows, select the most appropriate diagnosis.

(A) Adrenal carcinoma
(B) Congenital adrenal hyperplasia
(C) Cushing's syndrome
(D) Oat-cell carcinoma of the lung
(E) Nelson's syndrome

309. A 45-year-old man complains of severe weakness. He appears chronically wasted and is mildly hyperpigmented. His blood pressure is 160/100 mm Hg. Laboratory values appear in the table below. A high-dose dexamethasone suppression test (2 mg every six hours) causes no suppression of urinary 17-hydroxycorticosteroids (17-OHCS) or 17-ketosteroids (17-KS)

310. A 26-year-old woman complains of irregular menses, obesity, and low back pain. She has mild hypertension, central obesity, broad striae, acne, and mild hirsutism. Laboratory values appear in the table below. A low-dose dexamethasone suppression test (0.5 mg every six hours) causes no suppression of urinary 17-OHCS. A high-dose dexamethasone suppression test causes greater than 50 percent suppression of urinary 17-OHCS

311. A 20-year-old woman complains of weakness, easy bruising, hirsutism, and irregular menses. She exhibits a moon face, central obesity, and severe hirsutism involving the face and trunk, but no virilism. Laboratory values appear in the table below. A high-dose dexamethasone suppression test causes no suppression of 17-OHCS or 17-KS

312. A 15-year-old boy complains of short stature. He has a history of early sexual development and accelerated growth that ceased five years ago. He displays hyperpigmentation. Laboratory values appear in the table below. A high-dose dexamethasone suppression test causes greater than 50 percent suppression of urinary 17-KS

Laboratory Values

Patient Number	Serum K^+ (mEq/L)	Serum HCO_3 (mEq/L)	Plasma Cortisol at 6 P.M. (μg/100 ml)*	Plasma ACTH (pg/100 ml)†	Urine 17-OHCS (mg/24 hr)★	Urine 17-KS (mg/24 hr)‡
309.	3.0	35	40	1000	35	40
310.	3.9	25	20	90	15	15
311.	3.2	32	80	5	35	70
312.	3.8	25	13	250	4	65

*Normal: 10 to 24. ★Normal: 3 to 12.
†Normal: 40 to 100. ‡Normal: male <20; female <15.

Questions 313-316

For each case presentation that follows, select the lipoprotein disorder with which it is most closely associated.

(A) Hyperchylomicronemia (type I)
(B) Hyperbetalipoproteinemia (type IIa)
(C) "Broad-beta" disease (type III)
(D) Hyperprebetalipoproteinemia (type IV)
(E) Combined hyperlipoproteinemia (type IIb)

313. A 45-year-old diabetic patient complains of intermittent claudication. Physical examination reveals xanthomas of the palmar and digital creases and tuberoeruptive xanthomas of the elbows. Serum cholesterol and triglycerides are 320 and 280 mg/100 ml, respectively

314. A 12-year-old girl complains of acute abdominal pain. Physical examination reveals eruptive xanthomas, hepatosplenomegaly, and lipemia retinalis. Blood drawn on hospital admission looks like "cream of tomato soup"

315. A 32-year-old man has chest pain on exertion and a strong family history of coronary artery disease. Xanthomas are present on his Achilles tendon. Serum cholesterol and triglycerides are 380 and 150 mg/100 ml, respectively

316. A 24-year-old woman is treated with oral contraceptives. Routine blood studies reveal turbid plasma

Endocrinology and Metabolic Disease

Answers

254. The answer is A. *(Isselbacher, ed 9. pp 1750-1753. Tyson, Med Clin North Am 55:947-959, 1971.)* During the first trimester of pregnancy, diabetic women are particularly prone to hypoglycemia, a propensity that has been ascribed to fetal utilization of glucose and gluconeogenic substrates. Later in pregnancy, insulin requirements increase due to a rise in placental contrainsular hormones. In the patient presented in the question, diabetic nephropathy is highly unlikely because of the absence of proteinuria. Owing to the lack of evidence of estrogen deficiency on vaginal smear, hypopituitarism also is unlikely.

255. The answer is B. *(Ellenberg, pp 822-842. Isselbacher, ed 9. pp 1751, 2032.)* Diabetic neuropathy may involve peripheral, visceral, or autonomic nerves. Peripheral neuropathy leads to a bilateral, symmetric, predominantly sensory loss in the lower extremities and often involves the upper extremities as well. Sensory loss in the lower extremities may lead either to the painless dissolution of the ankle (or—less commonly—the knee joint (Charcot's joints)) or to weakness and atrophy of the intrinsic muscles of the foot leading to a painless plantar ulcer. Autonomic involvement may result in orthostatic hypotension, anhidrosis, vasomotor instability, or impotence. There is a striking correlation between impotence and neurogenic vesical dysfunction. Necrobiosis lipoidica diabeticorum is a disorder characterized by inflammatory and degenerative changes in the dermal collagen. The pathogenesis of the lesions, which usually occur on the shins, is not clear.

256. The answer is A. *(Isselbacher, ed 9. pp 1709-1710.)* Although well-differentiated thyroid carcinomas in women under age 40 behave almost like benign disease, these tumors are far more aggressive in the elderly, particularly in men. Cold nodules are far less common in men than in women, and the risk of carcinoma is higher. Thus, the physician should not attempt a trial of suppressive thyroid treatment for a 60-year-old man who has a cold nodule, but should refer him for surgery. In such a patient, a needle biopsy could cause the tumor to spread and so should be avoided.

257. The answer is E. *(Bondy, ed 8. pp 1663-1677. Isselbacher, ed 9. p 1740.)* Patients who have pheochromocytoma frequently demonstrate reduced circulating plasma volume, probably as a consequence of chronic, excessive alpha-adrenergic stimulation. Reduced plasma volume is suggested clinically by orthostatic hypotension or by elevated hematocrit. If plasma volume is reduced preoperatively and not corrected by infusion of plasma or treatment with phenoxybenzamine, severe hypotension may occur during surgery immediately after removal of the tumor. Hypotension under such circumstances is best treated with volume expansion (e.g., blood replacement) rather than with a vasoconstrictive agent.

258. The answer is C. *(Bondy, ed 8. pp 1214-1220. Isselbacher, ed 9. p 1676.)* The presence of normal gonadotropins in the face of severe testosterone deficiency indicates pituitary insufficiency rather than primary testicular disease; in the latter circumstance, gonadotropin levels would be markedly increased. Since the symptoms of the patient presented in the question are of recent origin, loss of secondary sexual characteristics and testicular atrophy would be expected to be minimal. Although testosterone treatment is indicated, failure to evaluate the patient for adrenal and thyroid hypofunction or the presence of a pituitary tumor would be a serious oversight. In diabetes or psychiatric illness, blood testosterone levels are normal.

259. The answer is B. *(Bondy, ed 8. pp 1759-1770. Isselbacher, ed 9. p 1833.)* In the circumstance of surgical failure to locate a parathyroid adenoma, determination of parathormone levels in blood sampled from the veins of the neck and thorax has proved useful. This procedure is particularly efficacious when the small veins of thyroid plexi are catheterized. The other procedures listed in the question are nonspecific and would not distinguish parathyroid adenoma from nonparathyroid pathology.

260. The answer is C. *(Bondy, ed 8. pp 361-364. Isselbacher, ed 9. p 1762.)* The history and physical findings in the patient described in the question strongly implicate insulin-induced hypoglycemia. Treatment with propranolol would have made the patient particularly prone to hypoglycemia by blunting the counterregulatory hormone response to hypoglycemia. The presence of hypothermia also is an important clinical clue to the diagnosis of hypoglycemia. However, even if the picture were less clinically obvious, any patient afflicted with insulin-dependent diabetes and coma should immediately be given a large bolus of glucose. A 5% dextrose infusion is not adequate treatment.

261. The answer is B. *(Gordon, Am J Med Sci 271:252-268, 1976. Isselbacher, ed 9. p 1749.)* The nonketotic hyperosmolar syndrome is usually associated with a blood glucose level exceeding 600 to 800 mg/100 ml or a serum osmolarity exceeding 350 mOsm/L or both. Blood ketones are, in general, only mildly increased. Extensive burns induce marked increases in counterregulatory hormones (glucagon, epinephrine, and cortisol), which, in conjunction with the large quantities of glucose-containing fluids that patients with burns receive, may precipitate marked hyperglycemia. Hypertonic glucose solutions used in peritoneal dialysis may cause severe hyperglycemia in diabetic patients, as well as in uremic patients without known diabetes. The glucose intolerance of uremia is further intensified by the reduction in glucose excretion associated with uremic renal insufficiency. Phenytoin (Dilantin) directly inhibits insulin secretion, and thiazide diuretics reduce insulin release indirectly by inducing potassium deficiency. Phenformin is associated with an increased risk of lactic acidosis.

262. The answer is D. *(Bondy, ed 8. p 359. Isselbacher, ed 9. p 1762.)* The case history presented in the question is classic for insulinoma. The predominance of exercise-induced hypoglycemia and weight gain are characteristic of this disorder. Affected patients may have plasma insulin levels within normal limits after an overnight fast and frequently have glucose intolerance after glucose ingestion. The failure of insulin to fall when fasting hypoglycemia develops establishes the diagnosis of hyperinsulinism. In contrast, patients having reactive hypoglycemia do not develop hypoglycemia with fasting. Although hepatoma and Addison's disease may be associated with fasting hypoglycemia, insulin values fall appropriately during a fast in these disorders.

263. The answer is A. *(Bondy, ed 8. p 1595. Isselbacher, ed 9. p 1786.)* Ninety percent of children manifesting sexual precocity show no organic basis for their condition. A familial history of this condition is sometimes obtained. Affected children have advanced bone age, adult circulating levels of estrogen and gonadotropins, and normal adrenal function. Despite the rarity of organic causes of sexual precocity, lesions of the hypothalamus or pineal gland, which are associated with gonadotropin secretion, and estrogen-producing tumors must be ruled out. Because gonadotropins are suppressed by tumors that produce estrogens, true puberty does not actually occur in such disorders. The McCune-Albright syndrome causes, in addition to sexual precocity, patchy skin pigmentation and polyostotic fibrous dysplasia.

264. The answer is D. *(Isselbacher, ed 9. pp 1707-1708.)* Toxic multinodular goiter occurs not infrequently in a patient with long-standing simple goiter. This is a disease of the fifth or sixth decade of life, and women are affected much more frequently than men. The clinical presentation differs from that of typical Graves' disease. Exophthalmos is rare, while thyrotoxic cardiac disease is extremely common. Resistance to the usual therapeutic dosages of digitalis is common. The treatment of choice is radioactive iodine and large doses, usually in excess of 20 μCi/g of estimated thyroid mass, are required. In order to prevent an exacerbation of thyrotoxic symptoms caused by the destruction of the thyroid gland and the release of thyroxine as a result of a radiation-induced thyroiditis, it is prudent to initiate therapy with antithyroid agents and administer the radioactive iodine as a definitive treatment only when the affected patient has become euthyroid. Propranolol is not required in euthyroid patients.

265. The answer is C. *(Bondy, ed 8. p 1389. Isselbacher, ed 9. p 1696.)* The patient presented in the question has a classic case of iodine-induced hypothyroidism (Wolff-Chaikoff effect). Normally, individuals rapidly escape the suppressive effects of iodine on thyroid hormone production so that circulating thyroid hormone levels are unaffected. However, patients who are exposed to neck radiation (external or radioactive iodine) or who have glandular damage (thyroiditis or Graves' disease) are at risk of hypothyroidism. The source of iodine in this patient is the lymphangiogram, a procedure that would be expected to increase the patient's iodine pool for several years.

266. The answer is C. *(Bondy, ed 8. p 1365. Isselbacher, ed 9. p 1821.)* For the patient described in the question, the markedly increased calcitonin levels indicate the diagnosis of medullary carcinoma of the thyroid. However, in view of the family history, the patient may also have a pheochromocytoma (multiple endocrine adenomatosis type 2). These tumors sometimes are associated with an excess of catecholamines. Before thyroid surgery is performed on this patient, a pheochromocytoma must be ruled out through urinary catecholamine determinations; the presence of such a tumor might expose him to a hypertensive crisis during surgery. The entire thyroid gland must be removed, owing to the presence of numerous small and possibly malignant adenomata scattered throughout the gland. Successful removal of the medullary carcinoma can be monitored with serum calcitonin levels. Hyperparathyroidism, while unlikely in this patient, is probably present in his brother. These multiple adenomata are not associated with increased secretions of trophic hormones from the pituitary gland.

267. The answer is D. *(Bondy, ed 8. pp 1273-1284. Isselbacher, ed 9. p 1687.)* Metastatic tumors rarely cause diabetes insipidus; of the tumors that may cause it, carcinoma of the breast is by far the most common. In the patient discussed in the question, the diagnosis of diabetes insipidus is suggested by hypernatremia and a low urine osmolality. Psychogenic polydipsia is an unlikely diagnosis since serum sodium is usually mildly reduced in this condition. Renal glycosuria would be expected to induce a higher urine osmolality than this patient has because of the osmotic effect of glucose. While nephrocalcinosis secondary to hypercalcemia may produce polyuria, hypercalciuria does not. Finally, the findings of inappropriate antidiuretic hormone syndrome are the opposite of those observed in diabetes insipidus and thus incompatible with the clinical picture in this patient.

268. The answer is C. *(Bondy, ed 8. p 1605. Isselbacher, ed 9. p 1786.)* The symptoms of masculinization (e.g., alopecia, deepening of voice, clitoral hypertrophy) in the patient presented in the question are characteristic of active androgen-producing tumors. Such extreme virilization is very rarely observed in polycystic ovary syndrome or in Cushing's syndrome; moreover, the presence of normal urinary steroid and markedly elevated plasma testosterone levels indicates an ovarian rather than adrenal etiology for her findings. Although hilar cell tumors are capable of producing the picture seen in this patient, they are very rare and usually arise in postmenopausal women. Arrhenoblastomas are the most common adrogen-producing ovarian tumor. Their incidence is highest during the reproductive years. Composed of varying proportions of Leydig's and Sertoli's cells, they are generally benign. In contrast to arrhenoblastomas, granulosa-theca cell tumors produce feminization, not virilization.

269. The answer is C. *(Bondy, ed 8. p 1461. Carpenter, Medicine 43:153-180, 1964. Isselbacher, ed 9. p 1822.)* Although the patient described in the question has features characteristic of Addison's disease, four of her findings are atypical, i.e., hyperglycemia, thyromegaly, diminished reflexes, and positive thyroid antibodies. Addison's disease is normally associated with hypoglycemia. Furthermore, the severity of the hyponatremia, unusual in uncomplicated Addison's disease (generally serum sodium remains above 120 mEq/L), suggests another basis for her water retention, e.g., hypothyroidism. The coexistence of diabetes mellitus, Addison's disease, and hypothyroidism has been termed Schmidt's syndrome.

270. The answer is D. *(Bondy, ed 8. pp 1598-1607. Isselbacher, ed 9. p 225.)* The failure of the patient presented in the question to respond to medroxyprogesterone acetate (Provera) indicates estrogen deficiency, while her ability to respond to estrogens rules out endometrial failure (e.g., Asherman's syndrome) as a basis for her disorder. Since patients who have psychiatric disorders and polycystic ovary syndromes continue to produce estrogens, they would be expected to exhibit both withdrawal bleeding after Provera and relatively normal production of gonadotropins. In the patient under discussion, a diagnosis of ovarian failure or premature menopause is indicated by the marked increase in gonadotropins. In contrast, patients suffering from pituitary tumors have reduced gonadotropins.

271. The answer is D. *(Isselbacher, ed 9. p 1731.)* For most patients with adrenal failure, the ideal replacement therapy consists of 25 mg of cortisone acetate in the early morning with a further 12.5 mg of cortisone acetate in the late afternoon. With complete adrenal failure, the lack of aldosterone secretion will require replacement therapy with a mineralocorticoid, 9 α-fluorohydrocortisone. This is an extremely powerful drug and it is seldom that more than 0.1 mg/day will be required. Cortisone acetate provides the most convenient and cheapest replacement therapy. Although cortisone is not a glucocorticoid normally produced by humans, it very closely mimics naturally occurring hydrocortisone. Physiological replacement requires the administration of 25-37.5 mg of cortisone acetate, or its equivalent, in divided doses. Autoimmune adrenalitis has replaced tuberculosis as the most common cause of adrenal failure. It was the destruction of the adrenal gland by tuberculosis that was described in such detail by Addison. In planning replacement therapy, one must consider both the hormones that are not being secreted and the diurnal rhythm, which is physiologically important and normally controlled by the responses of the adrenal gland to hormones secreted by the adenohypophysis. Physiologically, most adrenocortical hormone is secreted during early hours of the morning, whereas the lowest level of hormone is secreted in the late afternoon.

272. The answer is E. *(Isselbacher, ed 9. pp 1724-1726.)* Aldosterone increases the exchange of intratubular sodium for secreted potassium and hydrogen ions in the distal tubules of the kidney. Inappropriate aldosterone production, first described by Conn in 1956, will exaggerate these physiological changes so that progressive depletion of total body potassium will occur at the same time as increased sodium reabsorption expands the extracellular fluid volume. By a mechanism that is unclear, these changes in sodium concentration and extracellular fluid volume cause a persistent rise in diastolic blood pressure. The most common cause of chronic potassium wasting is the use of diuretics. Primary aldosteronism should be considered in patients who are not edematous and not receiving diuretics, but who have a persistent hypokalemia. The use of potassium-wasting diuretics in the treatment of hypertension makes it difficult to evaluate hypokalemia in patients with an elevated diastolic blood pressure. The initial step in investigating such a patient requires the cessation of diuretic therapy for ten days to two weeks and administration of potassium chloride supplements, followed by a re-examination of the serum potassium level. If the hypokalemia persists, then further tests to evaluate aldosterone secretion are required. An examination of plasma renin will reveal hyposecretion of this hormone, which fails to increase appropriately during volume depletion in the presence of an increased secretion of aldosterone. Intravenous loading with sodium chloride to deliberately produce a volume expansion will, in the presence of this syndrome, fail to bring about the normal physiological reduction in aldosterone secretion. If severe diastolic hypertension or cardiac failure is present, however, the latter test is dangerous and must be applied with great caution.

273. The answer is D. *(Isselbacher, ed 9. pp 1788-1789. Wortsman, Ann Intern Med 90:923-925, 1980.)* The galactorrhea-amenorrhea syndrome, in which amenorrhea, infertility, and galactorrhea occur, is often characterized by normal-to-high prolactin levels. Studies have demonstrated that cyproheptadine therapy reduced the prolactin level in many patients. Since there is evidence that serotonin stimulates the secretion of prolactin, the effects of antiserotonergic agents are not surprising. Preliminary evidence that cyproheptadine may induce menstrual bleeding and decrease galactorrhea has been presented, although the effect on fertility is not yet known. In the Stein-Leventhal syndrome, which is characterized by cystic ovaries, virilization, and amenorrhea, prolactin levels are not elevated.

274. The answer is E. *(Bondy, ed 8. p 1734.)* The clinical presentation of a bilateral pulmonary infiltrate, together with nephrocalcinosis, hypercalcemia, hyperuricemia, and normal phosphate levels, is typical of sarcoidosis. The absence of any bone lesion, together with a normal phosphate level, make primary hyperparathyroidism unlikely. Furthermore, in primary hyperparathyroidism the serum chloride is frequently elevated and pulmonary infiltration, together with reduced vital capacity and diffusion defect, is uncharacteristic. The other causes of hypercalcemia are not associated with this clinical and biochemical constellation. The mechanism of hypercalcemia in sarcoidosis is not fully understood. It is thought that the hypercalcemia results from increased absorption of calcium from the gut, secondary to exaggerated vitamin D sensitivity. The mechanism for the reduction in hypercalcemia that follows steroid administration is unknown, but it is possible that glucocorticoids may inhibit formation of active vitamin D.

275. The answer is C. *(Isselbacher, ed 9. p 1695. Werner, ed 4. pp 422, 446.)* Thyroglossal duct cyst is the most important anomaly of thyroid development. Excision of the cyst is generally indicated because of the cyst's propensity to infection. Infection may enter the duct if a communication persists with the pharynx through the foramen cecum at the base of the tongue. After an acute upper respiratory infection, the duct may become obstructed. The obstruction can lead to cystic dilatation, thereby making the lesion clinically apparent.

276. The answer is A (1, 2, 3). *(Bondy, ed 8. pp 1281-1289. Isselbacher, ed 9. pp 1679, 1686-1691. Miller, Ann Intern Med 73:721-729, 1970.)* The ability of the patient presented in the question to concentrate urine clearly is impaired. His response to vasopressin (Pitressin) establishes the diagnosis of partial diabetes insipidus, thus ruling out psychogenic or nephrogenic causes for his urinary findings. Patients who have some antidiuretic hormone (ADH) secretion generally respond to oral chlorpropamide, thiazide diuretics, or lysine-vasopressin nasal spray. The negative salt balance induced by the diuretic leads to a reduction in glomerular filtration rate and to enhanced proximal tubular water reabsorption. This results in the delivery of less water to water-impermeable distal segments and so to reduced water excretion. While both chlorpropamide and tolbutamide have antidiuretic effects when given intravenously, only chlorpropamide is effective orally. The efficacy of sulfonylureas in this patient probably derives from their ability to enhance the action of ADH at the renal level.

277. The answer is C (2, 4). *(Bondy, ed 8. p 1760. Isselbacher, ed 9. pp 1834-1835.)* Hyperparathyroidism is frequently associated with personality changes, ranging from lethargy and mild affective disorders to mental obtundation and psychosis. The intensity of the symptoms is related to the magnitude of the hypercalcemia. Pruritus, which may be intense in hyperparathyroidism, disappears following parathyroidectomy. Electrocardiographic changes generally are limited to a shortening of the Q-T interval. Moniliasis is associated with hypoparathyroidism, not hyperparathyroidism.

278. The answer is A (1, 2, 3). *(Bondy, ed 8. pp 1461-1463. Isselbacher, ed 9. p 1733.)* Addisonian crisis is characterized by symptoms that are suggestive of acute gastroenteritis, i.e., nausea, vomiting, and diarrhea. Dehydration and hypotension are unusually severe, and fever (not hypothermia) is usually present. Hyperpigmentation is an important clinical finding, but since the syndrome may have an acute onset, hyperpigmentation can be absent. Laboratory data demonstrating hyponatremia, hyperkalemia, and excessive excretion of urinary sodium (greater than 750 mEq/day) strongly support the diagnosis of Addison's disease.

279. The answer is D (4). *(Bondy, ed 8. p 1754. Isselbacher, ed 9. pp 1296, 1303.)* Hypocalcemia may occur as a result of vitamin D deficiency—as in malabsorption or rickets—or vitamin D resistance—as in renal failure. The mechanism of hypocalcemia in pancreatitis is uncertain. In malabsorption, rickets, or pancreatitis, serum phosphate levels are low. On the other hand, in renal failure phosphate levels are invariably increased due to the inability of the kidneys to excrete phosphorus.

280. The answer is B (1, 3). *(Bondy, ed 8. pp 1780-1785. Isselbacher, ed 9. pp 1860-1863.)* Paget's disease is characterized by excessive and abnormal remodeling of bone. The markedly increased bone turnover leads to elevations in serum alkaline phosphatase level and in urine hydroxyproline excretion. Serum and urinary calcium levels are normal; however, during periods of immobilization, patients afflicted with Paget's disease can develop severe hypercalcemia and hypercalciuria.

281. The answer is C (2, 4). *(Isselbacher, ed 9. pp 1749-1750.)* Hyperosmolar nonketotic diabetic coma, usually a complication of maturity-onset diabetes, can be precipitated by any event that causes volume depletion. Hyperosmolar coma is associated with a mortality rate exceeding 50 percent. Administration of potassium salts usually is indicated sooner in the therapy of hyperosmolar coma than of ketoacidosis owing to an acceleration of intracellular shift of potassium during treatment in the absence of acidosis. Although patients with hyperosmolar coma are not overly ketotic, the hepatic mechanisms for generating ketones are normal. Ketone concentrations in the starvation range, 4-6 mOsm/kg, are observed in many patients.

282. The answer is B (1, 3). *(Isselbacher, ed 9. pp 1592-1593, 1719-1726.)* Regardless of etiology, Cushing's syndrome is characterized by excess production of cortisol. Most cases are due to bilateral adrenal hyperplasia secondary to over-production of ACTH by the pituitary. Harvey Cushing originally suggested (1932) that the excess ACTH was produced by pituitary basophil adenomas, a condition that was designated Cushing's **disease** before it was recognized that pituitary basophilism was only one of the causes of the syndrome that would bear his name. Because tumors may be very small and elude detection, or not be present at all, the frequency of pituitary adenomas as the cause of Cushing's syndrome is uncertain. The 48-hour dexamethasone suppression test is still an important screening test, since the failure of suppression of urinary 17-hydroxysteroid levels to less than 3 mg/24 hours, or of plasma cortisol levels to less than 5 μg/100 ml, by this test is virtually diagnostic of the syndrome. The most common nonendocrine tumor that secretes ACTH is a small-cell (oat-cell) carcinoma of the lung. In this situation, or in patients with adrenal neoplasms, no suppression occurs after dexamethasone administration, since pituitary ACTH secretion is already suppressed by the elevated cortisol levels.

283. The answer is B (1, 3). *(Hamilton, Medicine 52:195-215, 1973. Isselbacher, ed 9. pp 1708-1709. Savoie, J Clin Endocrinol Metab 41:685-691, 1975.)* Thyrotoxicosis associated with decreased radioactive iodine (RAI) uptake has been observed in: (1) patients who are surreptitiously taking exogenous thyroid; (2) Graves' disease with iodine loading; (3) iodine-induced thyrotoxicosis (Jod-Basedow phenomenon); (4) struma ovarii; and (5) metastatic follicular carcinoma. While a few rare cases of thyroid-stimulating hormone-producing pituitary adenomas have been reported, in this condition RAI uptake would be increased. Oat cell carcinoma is associated with several ectopic hormone syndromes but not with thyroid over-production.

284. The answer is A (1, 2, 3). *(Bondy, ed 8. p 1734. Isselbacher, ed 9. p 1837.)* The association of hypercalcemia with sarcoidosis is often most striking in summer and, in fact, may disappear in winter. This fluctuation probably is mediated by the effects of sunlight on vitamin D synthesis. Characteristically, patients who have sarcoidosis, vitamin D intoxication, or malignancy demonstrate a fall in serum calcium after cortisone treatment (100 to 200 mg/day). Parathormone levels in hypercalcemic disorders not associated with hyperparathyroidism characteristically are low. Brown tumors are associated with hyperparathyroidism and represent areas of uncalcified bone; they are not observed in sarcoidosis.

285. The answer is B (1, 3). *(Bondy, ed 8. pp 1762-1764. Isselbacher, ed 9. p 1834.)* Although symptomatic bone disease is uncommon in hyperparathyroidism, affected patients with asymptomatic bone involvement may exhibit early x-ray changes, among the earliest of which are subperiosteal resorption of the phalanges and resorption of the phalangeal tufts. X-ray bone evidence of hyperparathyroidism elsewhere in the skeleton without abnormal hand x-rays is unusual. Osteosclerosis is observed in hypoparathyroidism, and pseudofractures appear in osteomalacia.

286. The answer is B (1, 3). *(Isselbacher, ed 9. p 1750.)* The earliest sign of retinal change in diabetes is increased permeability followed by occlusion of retinal capillaries with sacular and fusiform aneurysms. Two types of exudates occur: (1) cotton wool exudates or microinfarcts, and (2) hard exudates. A sudden increase in the number of cotton wool exudates suggests rapidly advancing retinopathy. Hard exudates are much more common than cotton wool exudates. These lesions are probably indicative of leakage of lipids, serum, and proteins through damaged endothelium.

287. The answer is A (1, 2, 3). *(Bondy, ed 8. p 1742. Isselbacher, ed 9. pp 1854-1860.)* In contrast to osteomalacia, which is associated with hypocalcemia, hypophosphatemia, and increased alkaline phosphatase, osteoporosis is characterized by normal serum calcium, phosphate, and alkaline phosphatase levels. Urinary calcium in both conditions is normal. Pseudofractures are characteristic of osteomalacia but are not observed in osteoporosis.

288. The answer is E (all). *(Bondy, ed 8. p 1546. Isselbacher, ed 9. p 1797.)* A patient who has Klinefelter's syndrome usually presents with delayed puberty, infertility, or gynecomastia. The testes are characteristically small and firm. Biopsy reveals hyalinization of the seminiferous tubules and Leydig cell hyperplasia. Plasma testosterone levels usually are low, but fall within the normal range in 40 percent of affected patients. Fertility is extremely rare in patients who have Klinefelter's syndrome and follicle-stimulating hormone levels are markedly elevated.

289. The answer is C (2, 4). *(Bondy, ed 8. p 1213.)* After Klinefelter's syndrome, Kallmann's syndrome (hypogonadotropic hypogonadism) is probably the most common form of hypogonadism. Affected patients generally have a selective defect in gonadotropin secretion, their other pituitary functions remaining normal. These individuals are characterized by delayed puberty, eunuchoid proportions, normal stature, and low testosterone and gonadotropin levels. The testes' small size but normal consistency usually distinguishes them from the firm, rubbery testes characteristic of Klinefelter's syndrome. Anosmia or hyposmia is a classic finding and results from hypoplasia of the olfactory tracts. The origin of hypogonadotropic hypogonadism is probably hypothalamic, since the luteinizing hormone (LH) response to LH-releasing factor often is normal.

290. The answer is B (1, 3). *(Bondy, ed 8. pp 1510-1515. Isselbacher, ed 9. pp 1169, 1172.)* Diuretic therapy and malignant hypertension often induce excessive secretion of renin leading to secondary hyperaldosteronism, a condition that may be distinguished from primary hyperaldosteronism by elevated levels of renin. Renin is characteristically suppressed in primary hyperaldosteronism. Aldosterone levels are normal or low in Cushing's syndrome; hypokalemia in this disorder results from excessive cortisol and deoxycorticosterone production. Excessive licorice ingestion may produce hypokalemia and hypertension due to glycyrrhizinic acid in the licorice. This mineralocorticoid-like substance expands plasma volume and reduces aldosterone secretion.

291. The answer is E (all). *(Isselbacher, ed 9. pp 1789-1790.)* Cirrhosis and uremia are among the most common causes of gynecomastia. Estrogen- and gonadotropin-secreting tumors and hypogonadism must also be considered as causes. In addition, exogenous estrogens, spironolactone, and digitalis may produce this abnormality. Gynecomastia occurs commonly during puberty, occasionally in association with hyperthyroidism, and after recovering from severe malnutrition.

292. The answer is D (4). *(Isselbacher, ed 9. pp 1707-1708. Werner, ed 4. pp 509-513, 592, 604, 636.)* Onycholysis, or distal separation of the nail bed, is observed in over 10 percent of patients who have hyperthyroidism resulting from either Graves' disease or toxic nodular goiter; it usually begins in the nail of the fourth finger. In contrast, pretibial myxedema and exophthalmos are virtually pathognomonic of Graves' disease and are not observed in patients who have toxic nodular goiter. Thyroid acropathy, almost always associated with a history of exophthalmos and Graves' disease, is characterized by clubbing of the fingers and toes, swelling of the subcutaneous tissues of the extremities, and subperiosteal bone changes without new bone formation.

293. The answer is C (2, 4). *(Isselbacher, ed 9. pp 1706, 1709. Werner, ed 4. pp 53-54, 79, 332.)* Propylthiouracil has been shown to inhibit each step in thyroid hormone synthesis, i.e., iodination of tyrosine to form monoiodotyrosine, iodination of monoidodotyrosine to form diiodotyrosine, and the coupling of iodotyrosines to form T_4 and T_3. In addition to its effects on hormone synthesis, propylthiouracil blocks the conversion of T_4 to T_3 in peripheral tissues. Over 50 percent of newly synthesized T_3 derives from conversion of T_4 rather than from glandular synthesis.

294. The answer is C (2, 4). *(Isselbacher, ed 9. pp 1686-1691.)* The response to dehydration provides the most simple and reliable way for establishing the diagnosis of diabetes insipidus. Fluid is usually withheld from 6 A.M. to allow the patient to be carefully monitored over a sufficiently long period of time. It is necessary to withhold fluids until stable hourly urinary osmolalities have been established. A loss of body weight of approximately 1 kg will usually accompany this degree of fluid deprivation. A loss of greater than 2 kg of body weight would be hazardous to the patient and fluid deprivation must be discontinued at this point. Generally, 5 units of vasopressin tannate in oil is given subcutaneously a few hours after dehydration is started, with serum osmolality being determined immediately before the injection of vasopressin and urinary osmolality being carefully monitored during the hour that follows the injection. Until recently, the most effective treatment of diabetes insipidus had been to supply arginine vasopressin, which has a duration of action from 4 to 6 hours and could be administered as an intranasal snuff. However, a new synthetic vasopressin, desmopressin acetate (DDAVP), is now the preferred drug for the management of diabetes insipidus because a single dose has a duration of action from 12 to 24 hours. A number of diuretics have been paradoxically successful in preventing the loss of fluids in diabetes insipidus, of which hydrochlorothiazide and chlorthalidone are the most successful. Ethacrynic acid, however, is not effective. The tranquilizer, thioridazine (Mellaril), can produce a syndrome of water intoxication with normal diluting capacity in patients with diabetes insipidus. Similar toxicity has been noted in patients who have required large enemas or who have drunk large volumes of beer. Other drugs that have been useful in the management of diabetes insipidus include the sulfonylurea, chlorpropamide, which has been shown to stimulate ADH release from the neurohypophysis, and the anticholesterol drug, clofibrate.

295. The answer is E (all). *(Bondy, ed 8. pp 1210-1212. Isselbacher, ed 9. p 1957.)* Enlargement of the sella turcica is characteristic, but not diagnostic, of pituitary tumors. Suprasellar lesions like craniopharyngiomas and aneurysms may extend into the sella, producing enlargement of the sella and erosion of its walls. In addition, cerebrospinal fluid pressure can force the subarachnoid space into the sella, resulting in enlargement of the sella and compression of the normal pituitary (empty-sella syndrome).

296. The answer is C (2, 4). *(Bondy, ed 8. p 1475. Isselbacher, ed 9. p 1723.)* Approximately 15 percent of patients who undergo bilateral adrenalectomy for Cushing's syndrome develop pituitary tumors that were not apparent prior to surgery (Nelson's syndrome); whether these tumors were actually present prior to surgery remains a point of speculation. Nelson's syndrome must be differentiated from inadequate adrenal replacement therapy, which will also produce hyperpigmentation. In either situation, circulating adrenocorticotropic hormone levels are increased.

297. The answer is A (1, 2, 3). *(Isselbacher, ed 9. p 1680.)* Hyperprolactinemia may result either from autonomous overproduction of prolactin by a pituitary adenoma, or from reduced production of prolactin inhibitory factor by the hypothalamus. Elevations in prolactin levels are associated with pregnancy, hypothalamic disease (e.g., sarcoidosis, tuberculosis, craniopharyngioma), hypothyroidism, and uremia. Drugs such as phenothiazines, tricyclic antidepressants, reserpine, and oral contraceptives also may produce heyperprolactinemia. Hyperprolactinemia may be present in the absence of galactorrhea, and galactorrhea may occur without hyperprolactinemia. Because oral L-dopa suppresses elevated prolactin levels both in the presence and absence of pituitary tumors, it is not useful in the differential diagnosis of hyperprolactinemia. Although prolactin stimulates lactation, it does not induce gynecomastia.

298. The answer is A (1, 2, 3). *(Bondy, ed 8. p 1734. Ellenberg, pp 457-458.) Isselbacher, ed 9. pp 1753-1754.)* Patients who are restricted to total bedrest or subject to stress will demonstrate glucose intolerance that is a consequence of insulin resistance. Furthermore, immobilization of young patients undergoing rapid bone growth can result in hypercalcemia and hypercalciuria. The hypercalcemia, in turn, will suppress parathyroid secretion. The severe pain and stress of a fracture, such as in the boy presented in the question, could lead to the loss of normal diurnal rhythm for cortisol secretion.

299. The answer is D (4). *(Isselbacher, ed 9. pp 1720-1722.)* While an abnormal diurnal steroid rhythm is a hallmark of Cushing's syndrome, it is a non-specific finding and also may be observed in stress, obesity, or depression. Similarly, the overnight dexamethasone suppression test, virtually always abnormal in Cushing's syndrome, also may be abnormal in obesity, depression, severe illness, or in association with phenytoin (Dilantin) administration. Victims of Cushing's syndrome, in contrast to normal subjects, characteristically do not show an increase in blood cortisol after insulin-induced hypoglycemia. Finally, the presence of normal urinary 17-hydroxycorticosteroid excretion does not rule out the diagnosis of Cushing's syndrome; up to 15 percent of affected patients have values within normal limits.

300. The answer is A (1, 2, 3). *(Isselbacher, ed 9. pp 1746-1749. Kreisberg, Ann Intern Med 88:682-683, 1978.)* Acetoacetate gives rise to a positive nitroprusside reaction, but β-hydroxybutyrate does not. Thus, if a high β-hydroxybutyrate/acetoacetate ratio (B/A) is present, the nitroprusside test may be falsely negative. The B/A ratio may vary in individuals and it is possible for the acidosis to be due almost exclusively to β-hydroxybutyrate. In this situation, the diagnosis of significant ketosis can easily be overlooked. Activity of the carnitine acyltransferase system of enzymes results in transport of fatty acids into the mitochondria after esterification to coenzyme A (CoA). This system is activated in uncontrolled diabetes.

301. The answer is A (1, 2, 3). *(Isselbacher, ed 9. pp 1710-1711.)* More than 95 percent of patients who have Hashimoto's thyroiditis demonstrate high titers of thyroglobulin antibodies, thyroid microsomal antibodies, or both. Extremely high titers are virtually diagnostic of the disease. Lower titers of thyroid antibodies may be observed in 50 percent of patients afflicted with pernicious anemia and in 20 percent of elderly women. Relatives of patients suffering from Hashimoto's or Graves' disease, as well as patients who have other autoimmune diseases, also exhibit low titers of thyroid antibody.

302. The answer is E (all). *(Isselbacher, ed 9. p 1711.)* Subacute thyroiditis is characterized by acute or subacute onset of asthenia, malaise, and pain over the thyroid that often is referred to the ear, lower jaw, or occiput. The disease is probably viral in origin; it frequently follows an upper respiratory infection. Subacute thyroiditis is diagnosed on the basis of an elevated erythrocyte sedimentation rate and a markedly depressed radioactive iodine uptake. Frequently, a high serum T_4 level is observed which, together with "leakage" of iodine from the gland, produces an elevated protein-bound iodine level.

303. The answer is C (2, 4). *(Isselbacher, ed 9. pp 1750-1751. Kohner, Metab Clin Exp 24:1085-1098, 1976.)* Diabetic retinopathy is the leading cause of incurable blindness in adults. Fifty percent of patients develop retinopathy within 10 years of the onset of diabetes and 90 percent within 20 years. The disease involves two major processes: (1) nonproliferative (background) retinopathy, consisting of microaneurysms, hemorrhages, and exudates; and (2) proliferative retinopathy, consisting of abnormal new vessels in a fibrous tissue bundle. Although proliferative retinopathy is the more common cause of severe visual loss, background retinopathy may lead to blindness by compromising the macula. Nonproliferative retinopathy characteristically waxes and wanes and may actually disappear; a small percentage of patients who have proliferative changes may experience spontaneous improvement. The efficacy of improved glucose regulation in diabetic retinopathy has not been established.

304. The answer is B (1, 3). *(Bondy, ed 8. p 1374. Isselbacher, ed 9. p 1708. Sterling, JAMA 213:571-575, 1970.)* The clinical and laboratory findings in the patient presented in the question are most consistent with "T_3 toxicosis." This hyperthyroid state is a result of overproduction of triiodothyronine in the presence of normal or slightly elevated thyroxine. Radioactive iodine uptake may be normal or increased. "T_3 toxicosis" is observed most commonly in patients who have autonomous nodules or who have been treated for Graves' disease. The diagnosis is established either by the presence of elevated serum triiodothyronine (radioimmunoassay) or by an abnormal T_3 suppression test. In the patient presented, long-acting thyroid stimulator (LATS) would not be present; LATS is observed in Graves' disease but not in the presence of an autonomous nodule. While thyroid-stimulating hormone levels would be suppressed in this patient, currently the assay is not sensitive enough to distinguish between low normal values of this hormone and hyperthyroidism.

305. The answer is A (1, 2, 3). *(Isselbacher, ed 9. pp 1746-1749. Page, Br Med J 2:687-690, 1974.)* Acetoacetate levels—in contrast to glucose, β-hydroxybutyrate, and free fatty acids levels—may actually rise during the first few hours of insulin treatment for diabetic ketoacidosis. Since Acetest tablets and Ketostix measure acetoacetate rather than β-hydroxybutyrate (the major blood ketone), such serial measurements of serum ketones do not reflect the blood ketone response to treatment. For example, total blood ketones, as measured by quantitative enzymatic techniques, may decline by 50 percent during the first few hours of treatment without a demonstrable change in serum ketones, as measured by Acetest tablets and Ketostix.

306. The answer is E (all). *(Isselbacher, ed 9. p 1682. Spark, Ann Intern Med 90:949-956, 1979.)* Bromocriptine, a dopaminergic agonist, has been shown to reduce prolactin levels in up to 90 percent of patients with hyperprolactinemia. Since dopamine is involved in the inhibitory control of prolactin secretion, use of a dopamine agonist has successfully caused inhibition of prolactin synthesis in conditions thought to be associated with dopamine deficiency. Bromocriptine has thus been useful in hyperprolactinemic states associated with galactorrhea, oligospermia, amenorrhea, and impotence. In the treatment of acromegaly, despite the fact that growth hormone levels have not been uniformly suppressed, affected patients have exhibited excellent subjective clinical responses to bromocriptine, as well as (1) reduction in foot size, (2) improved facial appearance, and (3) increased libido. Since growth hormone levels do not necessarily fall during bromocriptine therapy for acromegaly, it has been suggested that bromocriptine has a direct effect on somatomedin, independent of the effect on growth hormone. The mode of action of bromocriptine in acromegaly, however, remains to be clarified.

307. The answer is A (1, 2, 3). *(Isselbacher, ed 9. pp 381, 1746. Klint, Diabetes 19:747-830, 1970. Knatterud, Diabetes 24:65-184, 1975.)* The University Group Diabetes Program study, the largest controlled clinical trial of oral hypoglycemic agents to date, concluded that tolbutamide (Orinase) and phenformin incurred a higher risk of cardiovascular death than diet alone. Of patients treated with tolbutamide, 12.7 percent died from cardiovascular causes, as compared to 6.2 percent of patients treated by diet and insulin. Similar results were reported with phenformin. On the other hand, the comparability in cardiovascular mortality between placebo- and insulin-treated patients suggested (at least in cases of maturity-onset diabetes) that control of hyperglycemia did not reduce cardiovascular death rates. While the risk of cardiovascular death was increased in patients receiving oral hypoglycemic agents, overall mortality was not significantly higher than in the group subject to diet-control alone.

308. The answer is C (2, 4). *(Freinkel, J Clin Invest 42:1112-1133, 1963. Isselbacher, ed 9. p 1760.)* Hypoglycemia in the chronic alcoholic patient generally is a consequence of ethanol consumption rather than hepatic dysfunction. In fact, hypoglycemia is normal following alcohol ingestion if preceded by a fast of 48 to 72 hours. Ethanol inhibits gluconeogenesis by reducing both lactate and alanine incorporation into glucose. Consequently, only patients who are depleted of glycogen and therefore depend on gluconeogenesis for hepatic glucose production are likely to develop alcohol-induced hypoglycemia. Accordingly, this syndrome is observed in heavy drinkers who have been eating poorly, whether or not they have underlying liver disease. Alcohol-induced hypoglycemia is associated with an appropriate decline in circulating insulin; therefore, hyperketonemia is commonly present.

309-312. The answers are: 309-D, 310-C, 311-A, 312-B. *(Bondy, ed 8. pp 1464-1486, 1821-1827. Isselbacher, ed 9. pp 1682, 1691, 1721, 1727.)* Ectopic adrenocorticotropic hormone (ACTH) syndrome, as may be caused by oat-cell carcinoma, is characterized by hypokalemic alkalosis, hyperpigmentation associated with elevated levels of ACTH, and myopathy. The characteristic clinical features of Cushing's syndrome are generally absent, probably because of the rapid development of the disorder. Urinary 17-hydroxycorticosteroids (OHCS) and 17-ketosteroids (KS), as well as plasma cortisol, are markedly elevated; dexamethasone fails to suppress 17-OHCS even when high doses are given.

Cushing's syndrome (bilateral adrenal hyperplasia) is characterized by the loss of diurnal variation in plasma cortisol, elevated urinary 17-OHCS, the failure of urinary 17-OHCS suppression with the low-dose dexamethasone test, and greater than 50 percent suppression with the high-dose dexamethasone test. Plasma ACTH concentration is normal or mildly elevated and hypokalemic alkalosis is rarely present. Urinary 17-KS levels may be normal or increased inasmuch as they do not reflect the rate of cortisol production.

Patients who have adrenal carcinoma often display signs of excess adrenal androgen production that sometimes overshadow the signs of Cushing's syndrome. Plasma cortisol and urinary 17-KS may be dramatically increased; there is no 17-OHCS or 17-KS suppression even with the high-dose dexamethasone test. Characteristically, plasma ACTH is very low in adrenal carcinoma; in contrast, in Cushing's syndrome and ectopic ACTH syndrome, the ACTH levels are normal or increased.

Congenital adrenal hyperplasia results from a deficiency of one of several possible cortisol synthetic enzymes, the most common being 21-hydroxylase. Adrenal androgen production often is dramatically increased, while adrenal cortisol production may be normal or decreased. As a consequence of the excess androgen production, virilism occurs in the female and short stature is frequent in the male because of early closure of bony epiphyses. Urinary 17-KS levels are increased in congenital adrenal hyperplasia but are suppressed by dexamethasone. This feature distinguishes the disorder from adrenal tumors. Hyperpigmentation results from the compensatory increase in ACTH secretion.

313-316. The answers are: 313-C, 314-A, 315-B, 316-D. *(Isselbacher, ed 9. pp 508, 516-517. Stanbury, ed 4. pp 580-637.)* "Broad-beta" disease is characterized by the accumulation of remnants of abnormal, very low-density lipoproteins (VLDL). These remnants, displaying a mobility on lipoprotein electrophoresis between pre-β- and β-lipoproteins, present as a broad smear ("broad-beta band") between those two lipoprotein zones. On ultracentrifugation, however, the remnants sediment with VLDL. Plasma triglycerides and cholesterol are present in an approximate 1:1 ratio. The disorder is familial and associated with premature vascular disease. Planar xanthomas and tuberoeruptive xanthomas (confluent, eruptive lesions) of the elbows are virtually pathognomonic of "broad-beta" disease.

Hyperchylomicronemia results from lipoprotein lipase deficiency. This is a familial disorder that usually appears in childhood, producing recurrent abdominal pain, pancreatitis, and signs of extreme elevations of triglycerides. The chylomicron test will show a thick creamy layer on top and clear plasma below.

Hyperbetalipoproteinemia is inherited as a dominant trait. Afflicted heterozygous individuals generally develop ischemic heart disease before the fifth decade of life. Clinical features include tendinous and tuberous xanthomas, arcus corneae and, occasionally, xanthelasma. The presumptive metabolic defect in this disorder is a defect in β-lipoprotein removal.

Hyperprebetalipoproteinemia may be familial but is more commonly secondary to another cause (e.g., alcohol, stress, diabetes mellitus, uremia, obesity, glucocorticoids, or estrogens). In the case of estrogens, increases in triglycerides are secondary to increased VLDL production.

Gastroenterology

DIRECTIONS: Each question below contains five suggested answers. Choose the **one best** response to each question.

317. A 45-year-old woman with a long history of heavy drinking is admitted to the hospital because of weakness, anorexia, abdominal pain, and fatigue. On examination, she is found to have significant hepatomegaly, jaundice, ascites, and splenomegaly. Which of the following laboratory findings is LEAST likely in this patient?

(A) Greatly elevated serum γ-glutamyl transpeptidase
(B) Greatly elevated serum IgA
(C) Absent pre-β lipoprotein band with all lipoproteins migrating as a single wide band
(D) Smooth muscle antibody present in a titer of 1:100
(E) Hyperuricemia

318. IgA deficiency has been associated with all the following gastrointestinal conditions EXCEPT

(A) an increased incidence of *Giardia lamblia* infestation
(B) a marked increase in plasma cells in the lamina propria
(C) nodular lymphoid hyperplasia of the small intestine
(D) flat mucosal pattern
(E) diarrhea and malabsorption

319. A 55-year-old woman received 5000 rads to the lower abdomen one year ago for a pelvic malignancy. She now has blood-streaked stools containing excessive mucus. A barium enema at this time would be most likely to show

(A) a normal colon
(B) elevated serum IgA
(C) multiple polypoid lesions
(D) stricture of the rectum and sigmoid colon
(E) a fistula between the sigmoid colon and vagina

320. A 40-year-old man has symptoms suggestive of a peptic ulcer. An upper GI series reveals a small, apparently uncomplicated duodenal ulcer. In addition, there is marked rugal hypertrophy in the stomach and swelling of the folds in the duodenum. The next step in the evaluation of this patient should be

(A) panendoscopy
(B) gastric analysis
(C) assay of serum gastrin
(D) pancreatic function tests
(E) barium enema

321. Ulcerative colitis may occur in association with all the following complications EXCEPT

(A) ankylosing spondylitis
(B) arthritis of the large joints
(C) clubbing of the fingers
(D) erythema multiforme
(E) hepatocellular carcinoma

322. All the following statements about idiopathic hemochromatosis are true EXCEPT that

(A) the disorder is inherited as an autosomal recessive trait
(B) the disorder has an association with HLA-A3
(C) in untreated patients with clinically manifest hemochromatosis, serum ferritin level correlate with the magnitude of body iron stores
(D) in established cases, weekly phlebotomy reduces iron stores to normal within 6 months
(E) following reduction of iron stores to normal, phlebotomy is required every 3-4 months to prevent reaccumulation of iron

323. Inflammatory bowel disease has been associated with all the following hepatobiliary conditions EXCEPT

(A) chronic active hepatitis
(B) hepatoma
(C) pericholangitis
(D) sclerosing cholangitis
(E) amyloidosis

324. A 42-year-old woman who has stable, postnecrotic cirrhosis suddenly deteriorates, developing ascites, edema, and more jaundice. This deterioration is most likely to be explained by which of the following tests?

(A) Bromsulphalein test
(B) Smooth muscle antibody determination
(C) Serum 5′-nucleotidase determination
(D) Serum alpha-fetoprotein determination
(E) Blood ammonia determination

325. A 50-year-old alcoholic woman undergoes an upper gastrointestinal series to evaluate vague, dyspeptic symptoms and a loss of weight. She is found to have a small ulcer on the greater curvature of the stomach. The ulcer is sharply punched out, exhibiting radiating folds and Hampton's line. All the following statements in reference to this patient are correct EXCEPT that

(A) gastroscopy and biopsy should be performed
(B) gastric acid studies are useful only if absolute achlorhydria is found
(C) if the ulcer is benign, there is a 50 percent chance that it will heal in three weeks and a 70 percent chance that it will heal in six weeks
(D) if the ulcer is benign, a repeat upper GI series should be done at eight weeks with recommendation for surgery if the ulcer has not healed
(E) a history of alcoholism does not increase the likelihood of gastric ulceration

326. Intestinal calcium absorption is increased by all the following factors EXCEPT

(A) pregnancy
(B) systemic alkalosis
(C) low dietary intake of calcium
(D) corticosteroid therapy
(E) neomycin administration

327. A 22-year-old man is found to have a total serum bilirubin level of 2.5 mg/100 ml, with a direct fraction of 0.1 mg/100 ml. Other liver function tests are normal, and there is no evidence of hemolysis. The serum bilirubin level in this patient will undergo which of the following changes?

(A) Increase with phenobarbital therapy
(B) Gradually increase as he becomes older
(C) Increase during a 24-hour fast
(D) Diminish with high protein feeding
(E) Decrease after heavy exercise

328. Primary biliary cirrhosis is associated in 70 to 90 percent of affected patients with the presence in serum of

(A) hepatitis B antigen
(B) smooth muscle antibody
(C) mitochondrial antibody
(D) LE cells
(E) decreased $alpha_1$-antitrypsin

329. A 60-year-old man has diarrhea with blood in the stools and intermittent passage of clear mucus. On examination he is found to be dehydrated. Laboratory findings include:

Serum electrolytes (mEq/L): Na^+ 125; K^+ 2.2; Cl^- 85
Blood urea nitrogen: 60 mg/100 ml

The most likely diagnosis in this patient is

(A) familial polyposis of the colon
(B) lymphoid hyperplasia of the colon
(C) villous adenoma in the cecum
(D) villous adenoma in the ascending colon
(E) villous adenoma in the rectosigmoid

330. The incidence of colonic carcinoma is increased in association with all the following factors EXCEPT

(A) familial polyposis
(B) ulcerative colitis
(C) villous adenomas
(D) Gardner's syndrome
(E) Asian ancestry

331. A 42-year-old man is hospitalized for tachycardia. He has been having black stools for 24 hours. Physical examination suggests chronic liver disease. The initial diagnostic step should be

(A) aspiration lavage
(B) an upper gastrointestinal series
(C) panendoscopy
(D) determination of bromsulphalein retention
(E) arteriography

332. A 50-year-old man presents with a history of upper abdominal pain of six months duration. This pain radiates through to the back. He also has experienced a weight loss of 15 pounds over the same period, and jaundice of one month duration. On examination, he is found to have an enlarged gallbladder and to be moderately jaundiced. No other abnormalities are observed. Endoscopic retrograde cholangiopancreatography is performed and the result is shown in the x-ray below. The most likely diagnosis is

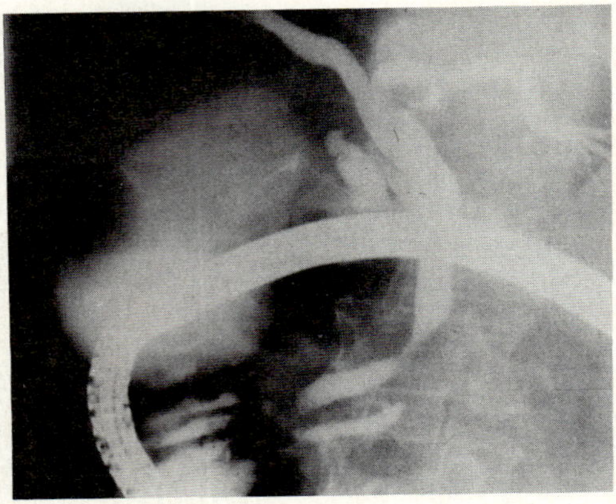

(A) choledocholithiasis
(B) chronic pancreatitis
(C) ampullary carcinoma
(D) pancreatic carcinoma
(E) none of the above

333. In an alcoholic patient, the clinical or historical finding that has the best prognostic correlation with the development of cirrhosis is

(A) liver biopsy evidence of alcoholic hepatitis
(B) the degree of fatty infiltration on liver biopsy
(C) the level of serum glutamic oxaloacetic transaminase
(D) the nutritional status of the affected patient
(E) the type of liquor imbibed

334. A 55-year-old man underwent surgery for benign ulcer disease. Several months later he began to complain of abdominal distension, pain, and weakness during meals, followed by faintness and headache. This patient should receive which of the following measures?

(A) Reassurance that his problem is self-limiting
(B) High-fluid intake at meals
(C) Multiple high-protein, low-carbohydrate feedings
(D) Insulin administration
(E) Oral hypoglycemic agents

335. A 55-year-old woman is admitted to the hospital for abdominal pain, recent onset of ascites and edema, and hepatomegaly; a diagnosis of Budd-Chiari syndrome is being considered. This diagnosis would be consistent with all the following findings EXCEPT

(A) high protein content of ascitic fluid
(B) elevated red blood cell and platelet counts
(C) serum bilirubin level of 12 mg/100 ml
(D) liver biopsy showing central venous congestion
(E) hepatic scintiscan showing excessive isotope uptake by the caudate lobe

336. A 35-year-old man complains of pain on swallowing both solids and liquids. The pain intensifies when he eats rapidly, although alcohol sometimes relieves it. Examination of this patient is LEAST likely to disclose

(A) enlargement of the colon
(B) air in the stomach
(C) manometric evidence of a high resting pressure of the lower esophageal sphincter
(D) a marked increase in lower esophageal pressure after giving methacholine
(E) termination of the esophagus in a beak-like appearance during barium esophagography

337. A 63-year-old woman is admitted to a hospital for jaundice. Liver function tests are as follows:

Bilirubin, total, serum: 12 mg/100 ml
SGOT: 250 IU/L
Alkaline phosphatase, serum: 300 U/L

The patient's transhepatic cholangiogram appears below. The next logical step in the management of this patient would be to

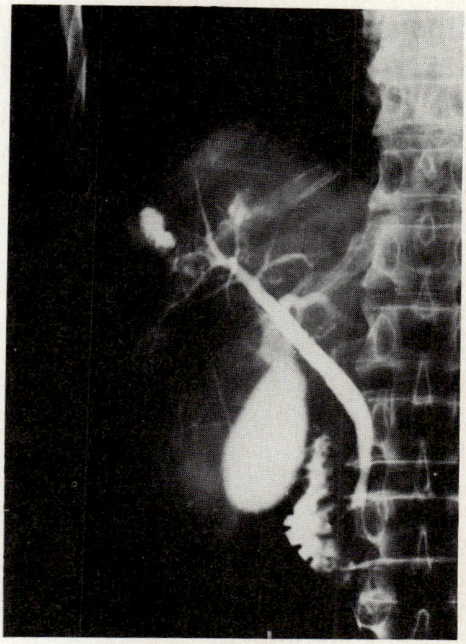

(A) perform a liver biopsy
(B) perform a laparotomy
(C) administer prednisone
(D) administer antibiotics
(E) perform hyperalimentation during continuous nasogastric aspiration

338. A 44-year-old man complains of colicky abdominal pain, dark urine, and light stools of one week duration. On examination, he is found to have moderate hepatomegaly, the hepatic edge being felt 4 cm below the costal margin. The gallbladder is not palpable, and there are no other abnormalities. Laboratory values are:

Bilirubin, total, serum: 10.4 mg/100 ml
Bilirubin, direct, serum: 6.9 mg/100 ml
SGOT: 90 IU/L
Alkaline phosphatase, serum: 270 U/L (normal 21-91)

The results of a cholangiographic study appear in the x-ray below. The most likely diagnosis is

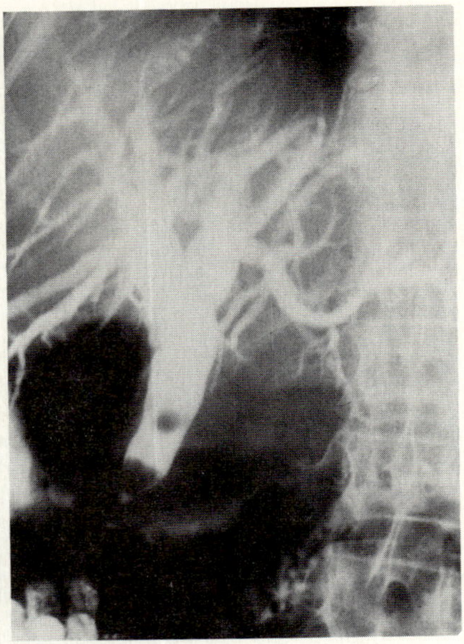

(A) carcinoma of the head of the pancreas
(B) carcinoma of the common bile duct
(C) carcinoma of the ampulla of Vater
(D) stone in the common duct
(E) stone in the cystic duct

339. A 21-year-old woman complains of having painful, stiff joints for several days. Physical examination reveals effusions of both knees and right upper quadrant tenderness. Laboratory data show a serum glutamic oxaloacetic transaminase of 1000 IU/l. The most useful diagnostic procedure would be which of the following?

(A) Liver scan
(B) Lupus induction test
(C) Serum rheumatoid factor determination
(D) Circulating hepatitis B antigen determination
(E) Arteriography

340. A 25-year-old woman complains of easy fatigability and malaise of several months duration. Liver function tests are abnormal and her serum contains smooth muscle antibody. Liver biopsy is reported to show chronic active hepatitis. Steroid therapy is begun. Which of the following results may be expected?

(A) Although clinical remission may be achieved, histologic abnormalities are irreversible
(B) Concomitant use of azathioprine will increase the incidence of steroid side effects
(C) Liver function tests will return to normal before the patient has symptomatic improvement
(D) If remission is attained, the chance of relapse following discontinuation of therapy is 50 percent
(E) Remission will occur only if steroid therapy exceeds 70 mg daily

341. A 45-year-old man develops dark urine, pale stools, nausea, anorexia, and right upper quadrant discomfort. On examination, his liver is found to be palpable two finger-breadths below the costal margin and is 2+ indurated (on a scale of 4) with a total span of 17 cm; the spleen is palpable below the costal margin and the abdomen exhibits shifting dullness. The patient indicates that he drinks three to four ounces or more of gin a day. In addition, he had eaten raw clams three weeks before the onset of his symptoms. For the past three years he has been taking alpha-methyldopa (Aldomet) for hypertension. Serologic screening reveals the presence of hepatitis A antibody (IgG), anti-HBs (titer: 1:16 by RIA) and anti-HBc (titer: 1:8 by RIA). Other laboratory values are as follows:

Bilirubin, total, serum: 10.5 mg/100 ml
Bilirubin, direct, serum: 6.7 mg/100 ml
SGOT: 94 IU/L
SGPT: 42 IU/L
Alkaline phosphatase, serum: 200 U/L

The most likely diagnosis is

(A) acute hepatitis A
(B) acute hepatitis B
(C) non-A, non-B hepatitis
(D) alcoholic hepatitis
(E) drug hepatitis related to alpha-methyldopa

342. A 60-year-old man known to have colonic diverticulosis presents with rectal hemorrhage, requiring a transfusion of two units of blood. Which of the following statements is most likely to apply to this patient's situation?

(A) Hemorrhage as a result of diverticular disease almost always is associated with inflamed diverticula
(B) Bleeding from diverticula usually ceases spontaneously and conservative management generally suffices
(C) Bleeding is relatively uncommon because the diverticula usually form on the antimesenteric border, away from the blood vessels
(D) Colonoscopy frequently fails to reveal the bleeding diverticula and is therefore not routinely done
(E) The presence of diverticulosis increases the likelihood of colonic carcinoma

343. A 35-year-old woman complains of weight loss and frequent, greasy, foul-smelling stools. She is observed to have thickened skin on her hands with ulcerations of the fingertips. Her gastrointestinal condition should be treated with

(A) surgery
(B) steroids
(C) azathioprine
(D) tetracycline
(E) gamma globulin injections

344. Following jejunoileal bypass surgery, all the following complications may occur EXCEPT

(A) polyarthritis
(B) diarrhea
(C) nephrolithiasis
(D) electrolyte imbalance
(E) chronic active hepatitis

345. All the following statements in reference to achalasia are true EXCEPT that

(A) dysphagia is present for both liquids and solids
(B) belching is often a major symptom
(C) vomiting rarely occurs
(D) absence of the gastric air bubble in a chest x-ray is frequently diagnostic
(E) manometry with the use of methacholine (Mecholyl) can readily confirm the diagnosis

346. A 25-year-old woman develops severe pruritus during the last trimester of her first pregnancy. She is mildly jaundiced. Within two weeks of delivery, both pruritus and jaundice disappear. All the following statements concerning this patient's symptoms are true EXCEPT that

(A) they will recur with subsequent pregnancies
(B) they usually occur throughout the course of a pregnancy
(C) they may be reproduced if the patient takes birth control pills
(D) they may have a genetic predisposition
(E) in the presence of symptoms, liver biopsy will show only mild cholestasis

347. Acute pancreatitis is best characterized by which of the following statements?

(A) The amylase/creatinine clearance ratio is usually less than one
(B) The degree of elevation in serum amylase is a relatively accurate index of the clinical severity of the lesion
(C) It is generally accepted that the development of a pancreatic pseudocyst is an indication for immediate surgical intervention with internal drainage
(D) Types I and V hyperlipidemias are predisposing factors
(E) Hypoglycemia, as a result of deficient glucagon levels, is a relatively common manifestation

DIRECTIONS: Each question below contains four suggested answers of which **one** or **more** is correct. Choose the answer:

A	if	**1, 2, and 3**	are correct
B	if	**1 and 3**	are correct
C	if	**2 and 4**	are correct
D	if	**4**	is correct
E	if	**1, 2, 3, and 4**	are correct

348. Non-A, non-B hepatitis is the most important form of post-transfusion hepatitis. Correct statements concerning non-A, non-B hepatitis include which of the following?

(1) Nonparenteral transmission occurs in a significant number of affected patients
(2) Anicteric hepatitis is as common as icteric hepatitis
(3) Gamma globulin given immediately after exposure has not been shown to reduce significantly the total incidence of hepatitis
(4) Chronic active hepatitis commonly follows this infection, has a more fulminant course than hepatitis B and has a higher long-term mortality

349. A 57-year-old man has clinical and histologic evidence of chronic active hepatitis. His serum is positive for HBsAg. Antigens/antibodies that are likely to be found by radioimmunoassay in the serum of this patient include

(1) HBeAg
(2) Anti-HBc
(3) Anti-HA(IgG)
(4) Anti-HBs

350. Budd-Chiari syndrome, a condition involving hepatic venous outflow obstruction, is characterized by

(1) a lower than normal radioisotope uptake in the caudate lobe of the liver together with increased uptake in the right lobe
(2) a frequently successful response to a side-to-side portacaval shunt procedure
(3) a histological appearance featuring peliosis hepatitis in liver biopsy specimens
(4) severe ascites that is resistant to diuretic therapy

351. Patients who have cholesterol gallstones exhibit which of the following characteristic findings?

(1) Hepatic bile that is either saturated or supersaturated with cholesterol
(2) Decreased total bile acid pool
(3) Decreased hepatic bile salt excretion
(4) In many instances, disappearance of gallstones in response to chenodeoxycholic acid therapy

352. Correct statements about primary biliary cirrhosis, a chronic disease characterized by progressive ductular damage, include which of the following?

(1) Gallstones are more common in affected patients than in the general population
(2) Penicillamine effectively limits both the degree of ductular damage and the development of overt portal hypertension
(3) Pruritus almost always precedes jaundice
(4) The female:male ratio of occurrence is about three to one

DIRECTIONS: The groups of questions below consist of lettered choices followed by several numbered items. For each numbered item select the **one** lettered choice with which it is **most** closely associated. Each lettered choice may be used once, more than once, or not at all.

Questions 353-356

For each of the gastrointestinal hormones listed below, select the action to which it is most closely related.

(A) Inhibits food intake
(B) Stimulates gastric acid secretion
(C) Stimulates pancreatic enzyme secretion
(D) Stimulates pancreatic bicarbonate secretion
(E) Stimulates hepatic glycogen formation

353. Secretin

354. Gastrin

355. Cholecystokinin (pancreozymin)

356. Glucagon

Questions 357-359

For each of the following sets of lesions, select the type of colitis with which it is most likely to be associated.

(A) Ischemic colitis
(B) Spastic colitis
(C) Granulomatous colitis
(D) Infectious colitis
(E) Ulcerative colitis

357. Skip lesions with rectal-sparing, perianal disease, fistula formation

358. Pancolitis, mucosal hyperemia and friability, colonic perforation

359. Mucosal engorgement, increased segmentation of distal colon, small-volume stools

Questions 360-363

For each of the diseases listed below, select the histologic picture with which it is most likely to be associated on liver biopsy.

(A) Eosinophilic globular inclusions in hepatocytes that remain para-aminosalicylic acid-positive after diastase digestion
(B) Eosinophilic perisinusoidal material that stains with Congo red
(C) Mallory bodies and balloon cell degeneration
(D) Acidophilic bodies and reticuloendothelial cell hyperplasia
(E) Bile duct degeneration with hyperplasia

360. Alcoholic hepatitis

361. Homozygous $alpha_1$-antitrypsin deficiency

362. Amyloidosis

363. Viral hepatitis

Gastroenterology
Answers

317. The answer is D. *(Isselbacher, ed 9. p 1451. Wright, pp 746-759.)* In all cases of alcoholic liver disease, γ-glutamyl transpeptidase is greatly elevated. This is a microsomal enzyme that is induced by alcohol. It may even be elevated in patients who consume large amounts of alcohol in the **absence** of liver disease. IgA frequently is increased in alcoholic liver injury and IgA:IgG sometimes is used to differentiate alcoholic from nonalcoholic liver disease. Smooth muscle antibody, however, is infrequently found in high titer in alcoholic liver disease and its presence suggests chronic active hepatitis. Pre-β lipoproteins are increased in fatty liver; in cirrhosis, the pre-β band disappears almost completely. Frequently, all lipoproteins migrate as a single wide band. Hyperuricemia is caused by a high NADH:NAD ratio with hyperlactacidemia. This situation may lead to secondary hyperuricemia owing to decreased urine excretion of uric acid and may account for the common association of alcohol abuse and gout.

318. The answer is B. *(Isselbacher, ed 9. pp 330-331, 588. Sleisenger, ed 2. p 60.)* Immunologic deficiency may be associated with several gastrointestinal manifestations, mainly diarrhea and malabsorption. Most commonly, the deficiency involves IgA, the predominant immunoglobulin present in the gastrointestinal cells that secrete immunoglobulins.

319. The answer is D. *(Isselbacher, ed 9. pp 942-945, 1427. Sleisenger, ed 2. pp 1736-1741.)* Radiation enterocolitis may occur in patients who have had radiotherapy exceeding a total dose of 4000 rads for pelvic tumors. The symptoms can occur at variable times in relation to therapy, often after several months. Early changes revealed on barium enema examination would include irregularity, spasm, and fine serrations of the bowel wall; after one year, of the findings listed in the question, examination would be most likely to reveal stricture formation.

320. The answer is C. *(Isselbacher, ed 9. pp 1382-1383. Spiro, ed 2. p 360.)* Edema and swelling of the gastric and duodenal folds, as well as gastric hypersecretion with marked rugal hypertrophy, are characteristic of the Zollinger-Ellison syndrome. Although the syndrome may present with markedly atypical ulcers, the most common presenting manifestation is that of an uncomplicated duodenal ulcer. The best current definitive test for confirming the diagnosis of this syndrome is a direct assay of serum gastrin. Normal fasting levels range between 50-200 pg/ml, whereas in the Zollinger-Ellison syndrome, serum gastrin levels usually are greater than 1000 pg/ml.

321. The answer is E. *(Isselbacher, ed 9. p 1885. Spiro, ed 2. pp 815-816.)* Ankylosing spondylitis has been observed in a significant number of patients with ulcerative colitis; the incidence of concurrence of these disorders is found to be as high as 30 percent in patients who have had ulcerative colitis for more than 10 years. Close relatives of patients with ulcerative colitis also have a higher incidence of ankylosing spondylitis than the normal population. Although sacroiliac disease with spondylitis also is fairly common in conjunction with ulcerative colitis, in most affected patients this lesion does not progress to florid ankylosis. Clubbing of the fingers also has been associated with ulcerative colitis, particularly if either the proximal part or large segments of the colon are involved. The association of ulcerative colitis with erythema multiforme is well described. Latex-negative arthritis, often involving large joints and often monarticular, is fairly common in association with ulcerative colitis. The joint symptoms frequently parallel the activity of the intestinal disease. Generally, joint disease is found more commonly in patients who have other evidence of extraintestinal manifestations of ulcerative colitis. Although the incidence of cholangiocarcinoma is increased in patients with ulcerative colitis, there is no increase in the incidence of hepatocellular carcinoma.

322. The answer is D. *(Isselbacher, ed 9. pp 488-491. Powell, Gastroenterology 78:374-381, 1980.)* The mainstay of therapy for idiopathic hemochromatosis continues to be routine phlebotomy. However, even in precirrhotic patients it will take between 18 and 24 months to reduce iron stores to acceptable levels. In older cirrhotic patients, the required duration of therapy may be longer. Usual treatment regimens include the weekly or biweekly removal of 500 ml of blood, a volume that contains 200-250 mg of iron. While this treatment initially may produce a mild anemia, stabilization of hemoglobin levels occurs within a few weeks and most affected patients tolerate the procedure well. In advance stages of hemochromatosis and certainly in those patients who have developed cirrhosis, at least 25 g of iron must be removed. Thus, weekly phlebotomies for periods of up to three years are needed in some cases. While iron stores are being reduced to normal, routine phlebotomy is arranged to keep plasma iron levels at approximately 150 μg/100 ml. Constant checking for the possible reaccumulation of iron is necessary. This determination is made by carefully monitoring plasma iron levels and the percentage of saturation of transferrin with iron. Changes in these indices will precede any increases in serum ferritin concentration.

323. The answer is B. *(Isselbacher, ed 9. p 1429.)* Inflammatory bowel disease is associated with a wide variety of hepatobiliary problems. Fatty infiltration of the liver is commonly seen in seriously ill patients. Inflammation in the portal triads (pericholangitis) is also common. Ulcerative colitis is found with a high frequency in patients who have sclerosing cholangitis and bile duct carcinoma. The cause of these hepatobiliary manifestations of inflammatory bowel disease is unknown.

324. The answer is D. *(Isselbacher, ed 9. pp 1484-1485. Sherlock, ed 5. pp 670-682.)* Primary hepatocellular carcinoma should be considered in any cirrhotic patient who is deteriorating for no obvious reason. Serum alpha-fetoprotein is markedly elevated in more than 50 percent of patients who have this tumor and is, therefore, a valuable screening test. The test must be interpreted with circumspection, however, since patients afflicted with benign liver diseases also may show mild elevations of alpha-fetoprotein when levels are measured by radioimmunoassay.

325. The answer is E. *(Spiro, ed 2. pp 292-305.)* Although most benign gastric ulcers occur on the lesser curvature, some do occur on the greater curvature. The observation that an ulcer on the greater curvature is sharply punched out and is associated with radiating folds and Hampton's line favors the diagnosis of a benign ulcer. Biopsy at the time of gastroscopy is essential in the evaluation of a gastric ulcer. Gastric analysis is useful only in determining whether or not a gastric ulcer in a **truly** achlorhydric stomach should be considered malignant and an operation should be carried out. However, the presence of acid does not exclude the possibility of carcinoma; a gastric malignancy may be associated with high levels of acid. Most gastric ulcers heal in six weeks; an ulcer that has not healed by eight weeks is an indication for surgery. Surgery in this circumstance is advisable both for fear of malignancy and because such ulcers tend to chronicity. Although gastric erosions and duodenal ulcers are more common in association with alcohol abuse, a history of alcoholism does not increase the likelihood of gastric ulceration.

326. The answer is D. *(Isselbacher, ed 9. pp 1827, 1846-1848. Sleisenger, ed 2. p 248.)* Calcium absorption is an active process that occurs most efficiently in the duodenum. The process is dependent on vitamin D, derived either from the diet or from skin exposure to ultraviolet light. Corticosteroids are effective in decreasing calcium absorption and often are used to correct hypercalcemia.

327. The answer is C. *(Isselbacher, ed 9. p 1455. Sherlock, ed 5. pp 249-252.)* Gilbert's syndrome (unconjugated hyperbilirubinemia) is a benign condition in which there is defective hepatic uptake of unconjugated bilirubin. The prognosis for affected patients is excellent. Fasting causes a marked increase in the serum bilirubin level in this condition, whereas phenobarbital therapy may restore the level to normal.

328. The answer is C. *(Isselbacher, ed 9. p 1476.)* Primary biliary cirrhosis is a disease of middle-aged women in which pruritus is the featured symptom. The serum alkaline phosphatase level is invariably elevated, and serum mitochondrial antibody is present in a high proportion of affected patients. The only other condition in which serum mitochondrial antibody occurs with any degree of predictability is chronic active hepatitis (10 to 20 percent of cases).

329. The answer is E. *(Isselbacher, ed 9. p 1433. Spiro, ed 2. p 850.)* Although many benign polyps may produce diarrhea and bleeding, the classic cause of serious electrolyte disturbances are villous adenomata. These tumors are soft, sessile growths with broad-based flat attachments. When a villous adenoma grows large enough, the secretions of its goblet cells may represent a significant loss of fluid and electrolytes. If the tumor is sufficiently distal in the colon, the fluid and electrolytes will not be absorbed. Therefore, the syndrome of significant electrolyte depletion, particularly potassium, is associated with tumors of the rectosigmoid. This syndrome is not associated with tumors of the right side of the colon, which is the site of fluid and electrolyte absorption. Lymphoid hyperplasia is a benign condition that occurs predominantly in children and does not produce the electrolyte abnormalities observed in the patient presented in the question. Familial polyposis usually presents between the ages of 10 and 40; this, too, is a rare cause of severe electrolyte disturbances.

330. The answer is E. *(Isselbacher, ed 9. pp 1434-1436. Sleisenger, ed 2. p 1784.)* In both women and men, the large bowel is the second most common site for cancer. Several diseases, including those listed in the question, are associated with an increased risk of colonic cancer. In addition, the populations of North America and northwest Europe have a much higher incidence of colonic cancer than do those of East Africa, Asia, Japan, and South America.

331. The answer is A. *(Isselbacher, ed 9. pp 202-205. Sleisenger, ed 2. p 222.)* Aspiration lavage is an extremely useful procedure both to localize gastrointestinal bleeding and to provide information for further diagnostic studies. If blood is found to be present, lavage can be carried out to clear the stomach for endoscopy. Esophageal varices are not a contraindication to passing a nasogastric tube.

332. The answer is D. *(Isselbacher, ed 9. pp 1362-1363. Spiro, ed 2. pp 954, 1076-1077.)* The clinical picture presented by the patient in the question, together with evidence of pancreatic duct obstruction and narrowing of the common bile duct shown in the x-ray, are characteristic of carcinoma of the head of the pancreas. Although chronic pancreatitis may cause obstruction of both pancreatic and common bile ducts, other evidence of chronic pancreatitis would be present, such as calcification and a beaded appearance of the pancreatic duct, which are not seen in the x-ray. Ampullary carcinoma would not be consistent with the relatively normal appearance of the distal part of the duct, since the obstruction would be at the ampulla, causing dilatation of both pancreatic and common bile ducts. Absence of a stone in this patient effectively rules out a diagnosis of choledocholithiasis, which in any case would be unlikely to cause obstruction of the pancreatic duct.

333. The answer is A. *(Isselbacher, ed 9. p 1475. Schiff, ed 4. pp 847, 915-917.)* Alcoholic hepatitis, believed to be the precursor of cirrhosis in alcoholic liver disease, is diagnosed primarily on histologic examination. If affected patients continue to drink, a high percentage will develop cirrhosis. Approximately 25 percent of such patients who abstain from alcohol will recover over a period of four to seven months.

334. The answer is C. *(Isselbacher, ed 9. p 1381. Sleisenger, ed 2. pp 950-952.)* The dumping syndrome may be a complication of any surgical procedure for duodenal ulcer, but is most common after a Billroth II anastomosis. The early phase of the syndrome, usually within 30 minutes of eating, results from the rapid passage of hyperosmolar contents through the anastomosis into the proximal jejunum. The late phase, generally several hours later, is attributed to hypoglycemia.

335. The answer is C. *(Isselbacher, ed 9. p 1479. Sherlock, ed 5. pp 224-230.)* The Budd-Chiari syndrome may arise from obstruction to hepatic venous flow at any point from the hepatic lobule to the right atrium. (Constrictive pericarditis may cause a similar picture.) The syndrome is strongly associated with clotting diseases, particularly polycythemia vera. Biochemical tests show nonspecific abnormalities, but the serum bilirubin level rarely exceeds 2 mg/100 ml. In chronic cases, the caudate lobe of the liver, which has separate venous drainage into the vena cava, is enlarged.

336. The answer is B. *(Isselbacher, ed 9. p 1368. Sleisenger, ed 2. pp 519-520.)* Achalasia is a motor disorder of the esophagus involving a failure of relaxation of the lower esophageal sphincter during swallowing. The flow of both liquids and solids into the stomach, thus, is impeded; in addition, there is failure of normal peristalsis in the upper esophagus. In this condition, the esophagus gradually dilates and becomes so patulous that it may occupy 25 percent of the width of the chest. The resting pressures will be very low. The cause of achalasia is unknown but it is usually associated with an absence of neurons in the myenteric plexus. Chagas' disease may produce the identical clinical syndrome; however, cardiac muscle and the colon usually are also involved.

337. The answer is A. *(Isselbacher, ed 9. pp 1493-1494. Sherlock, ed 5. pp 711-713.)* The cholangiogram illustrated in the question is normal, thus ruling out extrahepatic biliary obstruction as the cause of jaundice in the patient discussed. The next diagnostic step should be a liver biopsy. Therapy should be withheld until the diagnosis for this patient is established.

338. The answer is D. *(Isselbacher, ed 9. pp 1496-1497. Spiro, ed 2. p 954.)* A stone in the common bile duct is visualized on x-ray as a negative shadow on the cholangiography of the common bile duct. In addition, the common bile duct is dilated and a further obstruction is seen distal to the well defined circular lesion. The patient discussed in the question offers a typical presentation of a common bile duct stone; carcinoma of the common bile duct, the pancreas, or the ampulla would be unlikely diagnoses. A stone in the cystic duct does not cause an elevated bilirubin level of the order of 10 mg/100 ml and the filling defect in the common bile duct is further evidence against such a diagnosis.

339. The answer is D. *(Isselbacher, ed 9. pp 1459-1463. Sherlock, ed 5. pp 321-325.)* In the preicteric phase of hepatitis B, a serum sickness-like syndrome may occur in 10 to 20 percent of cases. The arthritis in the patient presented in the question is associated with circulating immune complexes of hepatitis B antigen and antibody. Serum complement is depressed, and hepatitis B antigen has also been detected in the synovial fluid of patients affected by this syndrome.

340. The answer is D. *(Isselbacher, ed 9. pp 1470-1472. Schiff, ed 4. pp 803-809.)* Recent controlled studies indicate that approximately 80 percent of patients having chronic active hepatitis will enter remission with steroid therapy (20 to 60 mg daily or 10 to 30 mg daily in combination with 50 mg azathioprine). The sequence of remissions is: first clinical, then biochemical, and finally histologic. For patients who relapse when therapy is discontinued, subsequent courses of therapy nearly always prove effective.

341. The answer is D. *(Dienstag, J Infect Dis 137:328-340, 1978. Isselbacher, ed 9. pp 1459-1467. Wright, pp 137, 596, 755, 837.)* Acute hepatitis A becomes increasingly less common with increasing age. Approximately 80 percent of urban adults over 50 years of age have already been exposed to hepatitis A and have IgG antibody to this antigen. It is unusual for acute hepatitis A to present with evidence of portal hypertension, like ascites, as early after exposure to possible sources of infection (clams) as is the case in the patient presented in the question. Moreover, the SGOT:SGPT ratio of greater than two virtually rules out any form of acute viral hepatitis. Acute hepatitis B is invariably associated with HBsAg and not with low titers of surface and core antibodies. The incubation period of non-A, non-B hepatitis following transfusion is 18-89 days. Although alpha-methyldopa is an important cause of hypersensitivity hepatitis, the history of the patient presented makes drug-induced hepatitis unlikely. A large, firm liver with splenomegaly and ascites in an individual who drinks significantly, especially when the SGOT is significantly higher than the SGPT, makes alcoholic hepatitis the most likely diagnosis.

342. The answer is B. *(Almy, N Engl J Med 302:329, 1980. Spiro, ed 2. pp 644-662.)* Hemorrhage from diverticular disease is a common occurrence; it usually arises from **un**inflamed diverticula. Nevertheless, rectal bleeding must not be attributed to the presence of diverticulosis until other possible sources, including inflammatory bowel disease, angiodysplasia, carcinoma, and adenomata have been carefully excluded, usually by colonoscopy. If patients do bleed from diverticula, however, the outcome usually is good. Spontaneous cessation of bleeding is the rule and only in rare instances will conservative therapy fail to stop the bleeding. The characteristically mild course of the disease probably is attributable to the fact that small vessels (less than 1 mm in diameter) are generally involved. Diverticula usually form on the mesenteric location of the bowel, purportedly through sites in the muscle coats made vulnerable by the entrance of blood vessels.

343. The answer is D. *(Isselbacher, ed 9. pp 1402-1403. Sleisenger, ed 2. p 292.)* Scleroderma frequently involves the small intestine, resulting in dilated bowel loops and intestinal stasis. Bacterial overgrowth commonly accompanies the stasis. The malabsorption of scleroderma often can be effectively treated with broad-spectrum antibiotics.

344. The answer is E. *(Isselbacher, ed 9. pp 415-416. Spiro, ed 2. pp 478-479.)* Polyarthritis occurs as a complication of jejunoileal bypass surgery presumably because of circulating immune complexes. Cholecystitis is a more frequent complication; it is probably due to the decreased bile acid pool that results from the malabsorption of bile acids. Fatty liver and even cirrhosis, often indistinguishable from that associated with chronic alcoholism, frequently develop in patients who have undergone jejunoileal bypass procedures. Although the histological picture of chronic active hepatitis is not seen in these patients, Mallory bodies, centrilobular fibrosis, and neutrophilic infiltrates are noteworthy. Diarrhea, however, commonly occurs in this situation, a condition that may be due to bile acid malabsorption, as well as to bacterial overgrowth.

345. The answer is B. *(Isselbacher, ed 9. pp 1368-1369. Spiro, ed 2. pp 57-59.)* In contrast to patients with an esophageal stricture, in whom often there is no dysphagia for liquids, patients with achalasia have difficulty swallowing solids and liquids. Belching, however, is very rare, because of the tonic state of the lower sphincter. Vomiting occurs rarely for the same reason. Absence of a gastric air bubble, a frequent occurrence in achalasia patients, strongly supports the diagnosis. Manometry is a useful means of confirming the diagnosis, especially when methacholine (Mecholyl) is injected; the baseline pressure rises sharply and suddenly and forceful waves may appear in the esophagus. In normal individuals, there is only a slight rise in the baseline pressure.

346. The answer is B. *(Isselbacher, ed 9. p 1457. Sherlock, ed 5. pp 573-574.)* Recurrent cholestasis of pregnancy probably is due to an unusual sensitivity to estrogens. The condition occurs during the last trimester of pregnancy. Although it recurs with subsequent pregnancies, this form of cholestasis is a benign one.

347. The answer is D. *(Bradley, Am J Surg 137:135-141, 1979. Pollack, Am J Surg 135:199-201, 1978. Spiro, ed 2. pp 1013-1042. Winship, Gastroenterol 73: 593-603, 1977.)* Although hyperlipemia, and particularly hyperchylomicronemia, may occur with acute pancreatitis, it is established that types I and V hyperlipidemias predispose to acute pancreatitis. Urinary clearance of amylase is markedly increased during acute pancreatitis, the amylase/creatinine clearance ratio usually being over 5; the reason for this is not entirely clear, although a defect in renal tubular reabsorption of amylase has been suggested. Pancreatic pseudocysts occur in approximately 10 percent of patients following acute pancreatitis. Although the management of pseudocysts is controversial, recent data indicate that internal drainage of a pseudocyst, before it has developed a fibrous capsule, has poor results. The danger associated with conservative therapy for pseudocysts is that of rupture. Therefore, indications for surgical intervention in a patient with a pseudocyst are (1) rapidly increasing size of the pseudocyst, (2) development of an abscess, or (3) persistence of the pseudocyst for a period of six weeks. Although rupture of a pseudocyst increases the mortality rate, the unsatisfactory results of immediate surgery suggest that observation for the first six weeks is in order provided that the complications mentioned above do not supervene. Hyperglycemia occurs in approximately 20 percent of affected patients, owing to an excess of released glucagon.

348. The answer is B (1, 3). *(Berman, Ann Intern Med 91:1-6, 1979. Isselbacher, ed 9. pp 1460-1461.)* Non-A, non-B hepatitis currently accounts for approximately 20 percent of sporadic hepatitis. There have been a number of reports in which non-A, non-B hepatitis has occurred without percutaneous exposure. Anicteric hepatitis is two to three times more common than icteric hepatitis. Current studies have not conclusively shown that immune serum globulin prevents the total incidence of non-A, non-B hepatitis if given after exposure. The only study in which a protective effect of gamma globulin was shown was one in which the gamma globulin was given prophylactically to patients receiving multiple transfusions during open heart surgery. Although the propensity to develop chronic hepatitis after non-A, non-B hepatitis is as great as, if not greater than, that following hepatitis B, the course of the disease appears to be milder than hepatitis B. According to one recent study, the course of non-A, non-B hepatitis appeared to decrease in severity with time.

349. The answer is A (1, 2, 3). *(Miller, J Clin Gastroenterol 1:251-258, 1978.)* In chronic active hepatitis, HBeAg correlates with the number of Dane particles and the infectiousness of the serum. It does not correlate well with the degree of activity of the liver disease, but is not uncommon in association with chronic active hepatitis. Anti-HBc is almost invariably present when HBsAg is detected in serum, whereas anti-HBs is not usually found by radioimmunoassay in the presence of HBsAg. Anti-HA (IgG) is found in up to 80 percent of affected adults over 50 years of age.

350. The answer is C (2, 4). *(Isselbacher, ed 9. p 1479. Wright, pp 1009-1010.)* Budd-Chiari syndrome is associated with myeloproliferative disease, tumors, use of oral contraceptives, and pregnancy. The existence of a fibrous diaphragm across the upper vena cava, which is one of the causes of the syndrome, is important to identify because it is treatable. Most affected patients present with a painful, tender liver and severe ascites resistant to therapy. Portal hypertension occurs late in the course of the illness. Liver scanning with technetium (^{99m}Tc) shows central uptake of colloid in the caudate lobe, together with reduced uptake in the right lobe. This pattern of uptake is thought to be due to the fact that the caudate lobe often drains directly into the inferior vena cava. Although therapy often is unsuccessful, side-to-side shunt has proved useful in a number of cases.

351. The answer is E (all). *(Isselbacher, ed 9. p 1490. Sleisenger, ed 2. pp 1286-1289, 1290-1291.)* Cholesterol gallstones result from a primary defect in hepatic bile formation. Livers of affected patients produce bile that is saturated or supersaturated with cholesterol. In the gallbladder, macroscopic stones are formed from the individual cholesterol microcrystals. Long-term administration of chenodeoxycholic acid will dissolve gallstones in 50 to 60 percent of affected patients; it is thought to decrease cholesterol secretion.

352. The answer is B (1, 3). *(Isselbacher, ed 9. pp 1476-1478. Wright, p 724.)* Approximately 90 percent of primary biliary cirrhosis cases occurs in women. The usually insidious onset is characterized by pruritus and fatigue. Jaundice is a relatively late finding. There is no effective treatment for this disease; corticosteroids have not been shown to be of use. Although penicillamine has been shown to decrease the amount of copper in the liver, there has been no success with this drug in the long-term treatment of primary biliary cirrhosis, nor is there evidence that penicillamine effectively reduces bile duct injury. Gallstones occur with greater frequency in primary biliary cirrhosis than in other forms of cirrhosis.

353-356. The answers are: 353-D, 354-B, 355-C, 356-A. *(Isselbacher, ed 9. pp 1371-1372, 1500, 1503. Sleisenger, ed 2. pp 1400, 1405-1406.)* All known gastrointestinal hormones are polypeptides. Their measurement is useful in certain clinical determinations, including the diagnosis and treatment of hormone-producing tumors. Gastrin is released from the pyloric glands of the stomach. In addition to its effect on gastric acid secretion, gastrin stimulates pepsin secretion and smooth muscle contraction. Serum levels of gastrin increase markedly in gastrinoma (Zollinger-Ellison syndrome). Elevated levels are also found in patients who have achlorhydria or hypochlorhydria.

Because of its effect on pancreatic secretion, secretin has been used to test for chronic pancreatitis. Patients afflicted with this disorder fail to exhibit a normal rise in the bicarbonate concentration of their pancreatic secretions after being given intravenous secretin.

Glucagon, secreted by alpha cells of the pancreas, stimulates both hepatic glycogenolysis and an increase in blood glucose concentration. This effect on blood glucose is probably responsible for the inhibition of food intake and gastric hunger contractions associated with glucagon.

In addition to its effect on pancreatic secretion, cholecystokinin causes contraction of the gallbladder and simultaneous relaxation of the sphincter of Oddi.

357-359. The answers are: 357-C, 358-E, 359-B. *(Isselbacher, ed 9. pp 1422, 1424-1426, 1431-1432. Sleisenger, ed 2. pp 1585, 1603, 1662-1663.)* The diagnosis of colitis is frequently difficult. This is particularly true of granulomatous colitis and ulcerative colitis; although each type has its own characteristic clinical, roentgenographic, and histologic features, considerable overlap occurs. Granulomatous disease affects the small bowel as well as the colon. Ulcerative colitis may be limited to the rectosigmoid area. These two colitides are most clearly differentiated by the presence of noncaseating granulomas in granulomatous colitis.

Patients suffering from spastic colitis (irritable colon) usually have constipation, with characteristic small-stool volume. All three colitides are chronic disorders of unknown etiologies, hence therapy necessarily is symptomatic.

360-363. The answers are: 360-C, 361-A, 362-B, 363-D. *(Isselbacher, ed 9. pp 338, 1462, 1473, 1488. Schiff, ed 4. pp 252-266.)* Some diseases have characteristic findings on liver biopsy. Amyloidosis first appears beneath sinusoidal lining cells as an amorphous, eosinophilic material that stains positively with Congo red. Amyloidosis involves the liver in 80 percent of affected persons.

In $alpha_1$-antitrypsin deficiency, para-aminosalicylic acid (PAS)-positive cytoplasmic inclusions appear in hepatocytes. These inclusions stain for $alpha_1$-antitrypsin with specific fluorescent antibody and apparently reflect the failure of the liver cell to transport this protein into the blood.

Mallory bodies are cytoplasmic inclusions commonly found in alcoholic hepatitis. Their origin is uncertain, but they appear to be altered proteins. These bodies, which are not specific for alcoholic hepatitis, also are associated with protracted cholestasis.

Acidophilic (Councilman) bodies represent dying hepatic cells that have rounded-up and become very eosinophilic. They are seen in viral hepatitis, drug hepatitis, and other hepatitides.

Diseases of the Urinary Tract

DIRECTIONS: Each question below contains five suggested answers. Choose the **one best** response to each question.

364. The most common renal neoplasm is a hypernephroma. This tumor is associated with all the following conditions EXCEPT

(A) liver function abnormalities in the absence of hepatic metastases
(B) pancytopenia in the absence of marrow metastases
(C) anemia
(D) thrombocytosis
(E) eosinophilia

365. A 63-year-old man develops urinary hesitancy and straining to initiate the stream. He has no other health problems. On rectal examination, he is found to have an enlarged prostate with a small area of induration. A needle biopsy discloses an anaplastic tumor of the prostate that is confined to the capsule. There is no clinical, radiologic, or other evidence of metastases. The correct staging and most appropriate therapy for this patient would be

(A) stage A: radical prostatectomy
(B) stage A: irradiation with 4000 rads
(C) stage A: irradiation with 8000 rads, followed by radical prostatectomy
(D) stage B: irradiation with 3000 rads
(E) stage B: irradiation with 6000 rads

366. The most common benign tumor of the epididymis is the

(A) lipoma
(B) myxoma
(C) fibroma
(D) cholesteatoma
(E) adenomatoid tumor

367. Which of the following statements concerning urethral valves is true?

(A) They are usually anterior in location
(B) They are an infrequent cause of urinary obstruction
(C) They are usually caused by chronic urinary tract infections
(D) They are frequently demonstrated by voiding cystourethrography
(E) They should not be resected transurethrally

368. A characteristic of Wilms' tumor is that it

(A) usually affects children over the age of five years
(B) most commonly causes gross hematuria as an initial symptom
(C) histologically reveals sarcomatous and epithelial elements
(D) predominantly metastasizes via the lymphatics
(E) is best managed by radiation therapy alone

369. In a man with isolated hematuria who has had an examination of the prostate and external urethra, the next diagnostic procedure should be

(A) cystoscopy
(B) retrograde pyelography
(C) intravenous pyelography
(D) renal arteriography
(E) renal ultrasonography

DIRECTIONS: Each question below contains four suggested answers of which **one** or **more** is correct. Choose the answer:

A	if	**1, 2, and 3**	are correct
B	if	**1 and 3**	are correct
C	if	**2 and 4**	are correct
D	if	**4**	is correct
E	if	**1, 2, 3, and 4**	are correct

370. Correct statements concerning testicular tumors include which of the following?

(1) They are uncommon in blacks
(2) They usually spread by local invasion
(3) They are more common in cryptorchid than descended testes
(4) They are best treated initially by trans-scrotal orchiectomy

371. Carcinoma of the urinary bladder is characterized by which of the following statements?

(1) It is usually an adenocarcinoma
(2) It has a higher than average incidence in heavy cigarette smokers
(3) It is frequently a metastatic lesion
(4) It commonly presents with painless hematuria

372. Ureteral obstruction may result from which of the following abnormalities?

(1) Retroperitoneal fibrosis
(2) Retrocaval ureter
(3) Ureterocele
(4) Carcinoma of the prostate

373. A perinephric abscess is an abscess that lies between the renal capsule and the perirenal fascia. In patients affected with this lesion, which of the following statements are true?

(1) The lesion usually arises *de novo* without predisposing renal disease
(2) When advanced, the lesion points over the iliac crest posterolaterally
(3) Abscesses arising from staphylococcal infections usually produce bacteriuria
(4) Excretory urography often shows advanced hydronephrosis

374. Correct statements concerning vasectomy include which of the following?

(1) Recanalization as a complication of a sperm granuloma has an incidence of approximately four percent
(2) Vasectomy is performed routinely at prostatectomy
(3) Urinary levels of FSH and LH are significantly altered after vasectomy
(4) Immobilizing and agglutinizing sperm antibodies appear frequently after vasectomy and persist in low titers for many years

375. True statements about urinary bladder tumors include which of the following?

(1) The majority of tumors arise on the posterior wall near the dome and thus are easily seen on cystoscopy
(2) More than half the patients with malignant tumors have carcinoembryonic antigen in the plasma
(3) A tumor that is missed on routine cystoscopy can be visualized in a subsequent examination using tetracycline and ultraviolet light
(4) Benzidine, *Schistosoma japonicum* infection, and aniline all are significant predisposing factors

376. Adult polycystic kidney disease is characterized by

(1) progressive renal insufficiency
(2) large multicystic kidneys
(3) increased incidence of cerebral aneurysms
(4) autosomal recessive inheritance

377. True statements about testicular tumors include which of the following?

(1) Approximately 30 percent of testicular tumors secrete chorionic gonadotropin
(2) Sertoli cell tumors are usually benign and are feminizing
(3) Testicular tumors are relatively rare in blacks
(4) The prognosis in patients with positive hormone titers is generally good

378. Impotence may develop as a consequence of which of the following factors?

(1) Abdominoperineal resection of the rectum
(2) Priapism
(3) Traumatic rupture of the urethra
(4) Unilateral nephrectomy

379. Tuberculosis of the genitourinary system is characterized by which of the following observations?

(1) Renal tuberculosis is, after the upper lobes of the lungs, the most common late-appearing localized tuberculous infection
(2) Tuberculosis rarely involves both kidneys
(3) In primary tuberculosis, tubercle bacilli may appear in the urine in the absence of detectable genitourinary tuberculosis
(4) Tubercle bacilli flourish in the renal medulla owing to the comparatively elevated oxygen tension in that part of the kidney

380. Malignant lesions of the penis are associated with which of the following disorders?

(1) Buschke-Löewenstein tumor
(2) Erythroplasia of Queyrat
(3) Condyloma acuminatum
(4) Paget's disease

381. Prostatectomy may cause which of the following complications?

(1) Urinary incontinence
(2) Retrograde ejaculation
(3) Urethral stricture formation
(4) Epididymitis

SUMMARY OF DIRECTIONS

A	B	C	D	E
1, 2, 3 only	1, 3 only	2, 4 only	4 only	All are correct

382. True statements concerning an uninhibited neurogenic bladder include which of the following?

(1) It may develop as a consequence of multiple sclerosis
(2) It may improve with the use of anticholinergic agents
(3) It is associated with increased urinary frequency and urgency
(4) It is best diagnosed by measuring bladder capacity

383. True statements concerning renal vein thrombosis include which of the following?

(1) In children it may be secondary to dehydration
(2) It occurs in conjunction with hypernephromas
(3) Its initial symptoms are hematuria and proteinuria
(4) It is rarely bilateral

384. Trichomoniasis is correctly represented by which of the following statements?

(1) It is a parasitic infection that only affects women
(2) It may have clinical findings similar to those of gonorrhea
(3) It may precipitate small intrarenal abscesses
(4) It is effectively treated with metronidazole

DIRECTIONS: The groups of questions below consist of lettered choices followed by several numbered items. For each numbered item select the **one** lettered choice with which it is **most** closely associated. Each lettered choice may be used once, more than once, or not at all.

Questions 385-388

For each of the following statements, select the type of urinary calculus with which it is most closely associated.

(A) Calcium oxalate calculi
(B) Cystine calculi
(C) Uric acid calculi
(D) Magnesium-ammonium-phosphate calculi
(E) Calcium phosphate calculi

385. They are commonly known as "infection stones"

386. D-Penicillamine therapy is often indicated

387. If pure, they are radiolucent on x-ray

388. They may cause a positive nitroprusside test

Questions 389-391

For each of the following statements concerning testicular tumors, select the neoplasm with which it is most closely associated.

(A) Seminoma
(B) Testicular carcinoma
(C) Teratoma
(D) All of the above
(E) None of the above

389. Orchiopexy before 10 years of age fails to prevent development

390. Normal human chorionic gonadotropin levels are characteristic

391. Megavoltage radiation of 2500-3500 rads is tumoricidal

Questions 392-395

For each of the following genitourinary disorders, select the syndrome with which it is most likely to be associated.

(A) Nail-patella syndrome
(B) Prune-belly syndrome
(C) Von Hippel-Lindau syndrome
(D) Kallmann's syndrome
(E) McCune-Albright syndrome

392. Renal tumor

393. Cryptorchidism

394. Hypogonadotropic hypogonadism

395. Ureteral dilatation

Diseases of the Urinary Tract

Answers

364. The answer is B. *(Isselbacher, ed 9. pp 1355-1356.)* Common systemic symptoms and sequelae of hypernephroma include (1) fatigability, (2) weight loss, (3) cachexia, (4) fever, and (5) anemia. Erythrocytosis occurs in about five percent of affected patients; it is probably associated with erythropoietin production. Eosinophilia, leukemoid reaction, thrombocytosis, and elevated erythrocyte sedimentation rate are also observed. Hematuria, usually microscopic, is commonly present. Patients sometimes demonstrate reversible liver function disturbances. These disturbances occur even when hepatic metastases are not present. Pancytopenia in the absence of bone marrow involvement, however, is not a characteristic feature of hypernephroma.

365. The answer is E. *(Isselbacher, ed 9. pp 1771-1772. Smith, ed 9. pp 290-297.)* Stage A carcinoma of the prostate is a tumor confined to the prostate that was neither suspected nor detected clinically, but diagnosed either at surgery or at autopsy. A stage B tumor also is confined to the prostate but is clinically evident on digital examination. The dose of irradiation that is curative for prostatic carcinoma is 5000-6000 rads; 3000-4000 rads is insufficient for cure, and 8000 rads is an excessive dose. Controversy exists as to whether radical prostatectomy or radiation is the treatment of choice.

366. The answer is E. *(Anderson, ed 7. pp 1028-1029.)* Tumors of the epididymis are uncommon. They may present as painless scrotal masses incidentally found on routine physical examination, but occasionally such tumors cannot be grossly distinguished from foci of epididymitis. The adenomatoid tumor has been reported to account for approximately half of all benign epididymal neoplasms.

367. The answer is D. *(Blandy, pp 641-645. Isselbacher, ed 9. p 1353.)* Urethral valves frequently cause urinary obstruction in the male. They are a congenital anomaly and may be suggested in the newborn by the presence of a weak urinary stream or a distended bladder. Excretory urography may reveal bilateral hydroureteronephrosis; voiding cystourethrography and cystoscopy will confirm the diagnosis. Urethral valves are usually posterior in location, and treatment consists of transurethral fulguration. Temporary supravesical urinary diversion may be necessary to drain the upper tracts.

368. The answer is C. *(Blandy, pp 392-398. Isselbacher, ed 9. p 1356.)* Wilms' tumor (nephroblastoma) is one of the commonest nonleukemic neoplasms of childhood. This renal neoplasm usually appears before the age of three years and usually spreads by local invasion and blood-borne metastasis rather than by lymphatic involvement. An abdominal mass is the most common presenting symptom. Microscopically, Wilms' tumor is characterized by epithelial and sarcomatous tissues. Treatment of affected patients combines surgery, radiation, and chemotherapy. Prognosis depends upon the patient's age and the stage of the tumor.

369. The answer is C. *(Isselbacher, ed 9. pp 216-217.)* Isolated hematuria is hematuria without proteinuria, cells, or urinary casts. It is produced by urinary tract bleeding from the urethra to the renal pelvis. Frequently encountered causes of isolated hematuria include (1) urinary tract stones, (2) neoplasms of the urinary tract, (3) tuberculosis, (4) trauma, and (5) prostatitis. Renal pelvic and ureteral lesions frequently cause hematuria. Thus, excretory urography should be done before cystoscopy, which is an invasive procedure. Renal arteriography is indicated only in the presence of an anatomic lesion, like a cyst or tumor. Ultrasound, although of use in disclosing a dilated pelvis, is less useful for detecting minor structural abnormalities.

370. The answer is B (1, 3). *(Blandy, pp 1203-1230. Isselbacher, ed 9. p 1592.)* Testicular tumors are most commonly of the germinal cell type. They may occur in either testis but rarely appear simultaneously in both testes. These tumors are more common in undescended than descended testes; it is unclear whether orchiopexy in fact diminishes the chances of subsequent malignancy. Initial treatment for most testicular tumors consists of orchiectomy via an inguinal incision. The need for radiation therapy, chemotherapy, or additional surgery is dependent upon the type and stage of the specific tumor. Metastasis from testicular tumors is usually by way of the lymphatics.

371. The answer is C (2, 4). *(Blandy, pp 774-781. Isselbacher, ed 9. pp 1356-1357.)* Carcinoma of the urinary bladder is generally of the transitional cell variety. It commonly presents with painless hematuria, which may be gross in nature. A high incidence of bladder tumors is reported in heavy cigarette smokers and in individuals exposed to certain industrial chemical agents such as benzidine, xenylamine, and 1- and 2-naphthylamines. Metastatic tumors to the bladder from another primary site are not common.

372. The answer is E (all). *(Blandy, pp 535-536, 589-592, 931. Isselbacher, ed 9. p 1353.)* Obstruction of the left or right ureter or both may have a variety of causes. Retroperitoneal fibrosis may involve the ureters by encasing them and causing subsequent obstruction. With abnormal development of the inferior vena cava, the right ureter may pass posterior to it, and obstruction with resultant hydronephrosis may result. A ureterocele, which is a ballooning of the distal ureter secondary to a stenotic ureteral meatus, may cause significant ureteral obstruction; a locally aggressive or metastatic carcinoma of the prostate can do the same.

373. The answer is C (2, 4). *(Isselbacher, ed 9. p 572. Smith, ed 9. p 163.)* A perinephric abscess usually is a complication of an advanced chronic renal infection. When it is advanced and of significant size, the lesion tends to point over the iliac crest (Petit's triangle posterolaterally). Anemia, leukocytosis, and accelerated sedimentation rate are usually found. Pus and bacteria, usually gram-negative rods, are often found in the urine of affected patients. However, if the renal organism is a *Staphylococcus*, the urine may be free of pus and bacteria. Excretory urograms may show delayed visualization, associated with pyelonephritis, but evidence of advanced hydronephrosis or calculous pyelonephrosis is commonly seen. At fluoroscopy, the involved kidney frequently exhibits an absence of normal respiratory excursions.

374. The answer is C (2, 4). *(Smith, ed 9. pp 507-511.)* The complications of vasectomy are infrequent. Recanalization as a complication of the formation of a sperm granuloma occurs in about 0.5 percent of vasectomized individuals. Congestive epididymitis and transient local pain may be seen with variable frequency. Levels of serum testosterone and urinary FSH and LH are unchanged following the operation.

375. The answer is A (1, 2, 3). *(Isselbacher, ed 9. pp 907-908, 1356. Smith, ed 9. pp 278-284.)* The majority of urinary bladder tumors arise at the base and may involve one or both ureteral orifices or the bladder neck. Therefore, hydroureteronephrosis and pyelonephritis are common complications. Carcinoembryonic antigen has been found in plasma and urine in up to 70 percent of patients with malignant tumors. In the rare event that a tumor is missed on cystoscopy, tetracycline and ultraviolet light will aid in its detection. Although benzidine and aniline, together with other industrial aromatic amines, are associated with a high incidence of bladder tumors, infection with *Schistosoma japonicum*, in contrast to schistosomiasis haematobia and schistosomiasis mansoni, does not involve the urinary tract. Ova are deposited in the intestinal wall and not in the bladder. It is common for *Schistosoma haematobium* eggs, and occasionally those of *S. mansoni*, to be passed in the urine.

376. The answer is A (1, 2, 3). *(Hepinstall, ed 2. pp 89-92. Isselbacher, ed 9. pp 1343-1344.)* Polycystic renal disease is generally divided into the adult and infantile forms. The latter is often associated with cysts of the liver and spleen, and death in the neonatal period is not unusual. The adult type commonly becomes manifest after the age of 30; affected individuals may present with flank pain and hematuria. Work-up of patients in whom polycystic disease is suspected may reveal markedly enlarged kidneys and hypertension; renal insufficiency commonly ensues. General treatment should be directed to control of the hypertension and management of the renal insufficiency. Death from rupture of cerebral aneurysms occurs in approximately 10 percent of affected patients. Whereas the infantile form is inherited as an autosomal recessive trait, the adult familial form is an autosomal dominant trait.

377. The answer is A (1, 2, 3). *(Isselbacher, ed 9. pp 1592, 1772. Smith, ed 9. pp 298-303.)* Testicular tumors account for approximately 0.5 percent of all malignancies in men and 4 percent of all tumors affecting the genitourinary tract. The frequency of these tumors among blacks is lower than among whites. Types of testicular tumors include (1) totipotent cell pattern tumors, (2) interstitial cell tumors, (3) Sertoli's cell tumors, and (4) germinal cell tumors. Approximately 30 percent of these tumors secrete chorionic gonadotropin; the prognosis in those patients with positive hormone titers is relatively poor. Usually these tumors have a carcinomatous pattern. Sertoli's cell tumors are feminizing and present with striking gynecomastia; they are relatively rare in childhood.

378. The answer is A (1, 2, 3). *(Blandy, pp 954-962, 1072-1077, 1245-1246. Isselbacher, ed 9. pp 230-232.)* Although many cases of impotence are psychogenic, possible organic causes must be carefully ruled out. Interruption of the sacral parasympathetic nerves (S2-S4) may result from wide dissection in radical pelvic procedures such as radical prostatectomy and abdominoperineal resection, with resultant impotence. Fibrosis of the cavernous septa may follow priapism and cause impotence. After traumatic urethral injuries, vascular or neurologic deficits may compromise erection.

379. The answer is B (1, 3). *(Isselbacher, ed 9. p 705.)* Renal tuberculosis is caused by hematogenous spread of tubercle bacilli. With the exception of the upper lobes of the lungs, the kidneys are the commonest site for late-appearing localized tuberculosis. Although the infection may commence as a unilateral lesion, it usually spreads to the opposite kidney and to the urinary tract. The lesion usually is found near the junction of the cortex and medulla; in the cortex it is the primary site for growth of the bacteria. Approximately 10 percent of the patients with primary tuberculosis excrete tubercle bacilli in the urine even without any detectable urinary tract lesions.

380. The answer is C (2, 4). *(Blandy, pp 1054-1058. Harrison, ed 4. pp 1172-1175.)* It is important to distinguish benign and malignant tumors of the penis. The malignant group includes squamous cell carcinomas, sarcomas, and melanomas, as well as Paget's disease and erythroplasia of Queyrat. Paget's disease and erythroplasia of Queyrat are considered in situ carcinomas and have distinct histologic features. Condylomata acuminata are friable, papillary lesions known as venereal warts and are not malignant. The Buschke-Löewenstein tumor, which often resembles a large condyloma acuminatum, is noninvasive and may be controlled with local fulguration or excision.

381. The answer is E (all). *(Harrison, ed 4. pp 684, 1658, 1667, 1940.)* By whatever method, prostatectomy may lead to a number of complications. Urinary incontinence secondary to external sphincter injury may be devastating. Retrograde ejaculation secondary to resection of the vesical neck is very common and may produce sterility. Urethral stricture formation may result from faulty surgical technique such as inadequate lubrication, prolonged instrumentation, or use of oversized instruments. Epididymitis may also develop; it can be unilateral or bilateral, and its incidence may be lessened by performing a vasectomy prior to prostatectomy.

382. The answer is A (1, 2, 3). *(Harrison, ed 4. pp 1217, 1220, 1249. Isselbacher, ed 9. p 1328.)* The uninhibited neurogenic bladder is usually the result of impairment of the corticoregulatory pathways controlling urination; this impairment, in turn, may have its origin in multiple sclerosis, spinal cord tumors, or trauma. Symptoms of an uninhibited neurogenic bladder include (1) increased urinary frequency and urgency, and (2) incontinence. Cystometrography is useful in establishing the diagnosis, and anticholinergic agents may help in controlling the symptoms of this disorder. The finding of a small bladder capacity is not diagnostic of uninhibited neurogenic bladder, as several other conditions can cause diminished capacity.

383. The answer is A (1, 2, 3). *(Blandy, pp 362-365. Isselbacher, ed 9. pp 1341-1342.)* Renal vein thrombosis may be secondary to a variety of causes. In children, dehydration from diarrhea and vomiting associated with gastroenteritis may precipitate renal vein thrombosis. Renal tumors (hypernephromas) may invade the renal veins and result in thrombosis. The thrombotic process, which frequently is heralded by flank pain, hematuria and proteinuria, may affect both kidneys. Treatment of this disorder may include anticoagulation therapy, thrombectomy, and nephrectomy—if the process is unilateral.

384. The answer is C (2, 4). *(Blandy, pp 997-999. Isselbacher, ed 9. p 887.)* *Trichomonas vaginalis*, a parasite, is a common cause of vaginitis and can be transmitted by sexual contact. Trichomoniasis can cause cervicitis and urethritis, as well as vaginitis, in women and, thus, must be distinguished from gonorrhea. Urethral itching and discharge may occur in infected men. Treatment of both sexually involved partners with metronidazole (Flagyl) is usually quite effective. Renal abnormalities associated with trichomoniasis have not been reported.

385-388. The answers are: 385-D, 386-B, 387-C, 388-B. *(Blandy, pp 291-314. Isselbacher, ed 9. pp 1349-1350.)* Urinary stone disease is a common urologic problem involving many types of calculi. The relative incidence of these different types is related to such considerations as environment, underlying disease processes, and endogenous factors. Five kinds of stones are generally encountered. Calcium oxalate stones are very common, and are usually radiopaque on x-ray. High-fluid intake, dietary restriction of calcium and oxalate, and the use of thiazides and inorganic phosphate all have been reported to be fairly successful in controlling recurrent calcium oxalate stone formation.

Calcium phosphate stones are also relatively common and may be associated with hyperparathyroidism and renal tubular acidosis.

Uric acid stones are radiolucent on x-ray. Consequently, at times they must be distinguished from urothelial tumors. Dietary restriction of protein, as well as alkalinization of the urine, may be helpful in treating these calculi.

Ammoniomagnesium phosphate stones, also known as struvite, or "infection," stones are commonly associated with chronic urinary tract infections. Dietary controls have little effect on such calculi.

Cystine stones occur in individuals who have an inherited defect in reabsorption of cystine. Increased fluid intake, dietary restriction of protein, and the use of D-penicillamine (which binds to cystine and increases its solubility) may be effective in controlling recurrent cystine stone formation. The nitroprusside test is used to detect abnormal amounts of urinary cystine.

389-391. The answers are: 389-E, 390-A, 391-A. *(Anderson, Ann Intern Med 90:373-385, 1979.)* Testicular tumors are more common in the white population than in the other races—the only known other predisposition is a history of cryptorchidism. Orchiopexy after 6 years of age appears not to prevent subsequent development of malignancy in the involved testis.

Human chorionic gonadotropin (HGC) is a glycoprotein with a molecular weight of 45,000. Normal persons have serum levels of HGC below 1 ng/ml. All patients with benign disorders have normal HGC levels; approximately 70 percent of patients with testicular nonseminomatous germ cell tumors have elevated HGC levels. Therefore, patients with both testicular carcinoma and teratoma may have elevated HGC levels but patients with seminoma do not.

A dose of 2500-3500 rads is usually tumoricidal for seminoma. Generally, this dose effectively kills tumor cells. The dose required for embryonal carcinoma is in excess of 4500 rads.

392-395. The answers are: 392-C, 393-B, 394-D, 395-B. *(Isselbacher, ed 9. pp 1808, 2007, 2021. Vaughan, ed 11. pp 1766, 1951.)* Many pediatric syndromes have associated genitourinary abnormalities. Prune-belly syndrome is characterized by (1) varying degrees of deficiency in abdominal musculature, (2) ureteral dilatation, and (3) undescended testes. Other anomalies such as urethral valves may be present. It is thought that the abnormal abdominal musculature results in weak intra-abdominal pressure that—along with the presence of adequate amounts of androgens—is necessary for the proper descent of the testicles to their normal scrotal position.

Retinal and cerebellar angiomas, renal tumors or cysts, and pancreatic cysts are features of the Von Hippel-Lindau syndrome. Although the inheritance of the disease is variable, most cases appear to be transmitted as an autosomal dominant defect, but many cases arise sporadically. The tumors usually begin after puberty. The retinal lesion described by Von Hippel is not always associated with the full syndrome. Other tumors that have been reported include pheochromocytomas, hemangioblastomas (spinal hemangioblastomas producing the syndrome of syringomyelia), and associated cerebellar hemangioblastomas frequently presenting as the cerebellar tumor syndrome.

Hypogonadism—secondary to a deficiency in gonadotropins—and anosmia—secondary to agenesis of the olfactory lobes—characterize Kallmann's syndrome.

Individuals who have the McCune-Albright syndrome demonstrate precocious puberty.

Oncology and Hematology

DIRECTIONS: Each question below contains five suggested answers. Choose the **one best** response to each question.

396. A 20-year-old college student seeks medical attention because of a fever of 38.9°C (102°F) and a weight loss of 9 kg (20 pounds) in two months. On physical examination, she is found to have enlarged cervical, supraclavicular, and axillary nodes. No nodes are palpable below the diaphragm and there is no organomegaly. Chest x-ray reveals hilar adenopathy, and tomography reveals extension of the pathologic process into the adjacent perihilar pulmonary parenchyma. Biopsy of a cervical node reveals nodular sclerosing Hodgkin's disease. A retroperitoneal lymphangiogram is unequivocally abnormal. The clinical stage (CS) at this point is

(A) CS IIB_E
(B) CS IIIB
(C) CS $IIIB_E$
(D) CS $IIIB_{ES}$
(E) CS IVB

397. A 55-year-old man undergoes a partial gastrectomy for a duodenal ulcer. Two years after gastrectomy he complains of easy fatigability and dyspnea. On examination, the sole abnormality is pale oral mucosa. The LEAST likely hematological finding in this patient would be which of the following?

(A) Mean corpuscular volume of 104 μm^3
(B) Anisocytosis with numerous macroovalocytes
(C) Basophilic stippling
(D) Marked increase in lactic acid dehydrogenase (isoenzyme 1)
(E) Vitamin B_{12} plasma level of 300 pg/ml

398. A 40-year-old woman, who had a mastectomy for adenocarcinoma of the breast a year ago, now complains of anorexia, weight loss, and dull ache in the right upper quadrant. She has regular menses. On physical examination, the patient is found to have an enlarged, nodular liver; biopsy discloses adenocarcinoma. The treatment of choice would be

(A) bilateral oophorectomy
(B) hepatic irradiation
(C) administration of diethylstilbestrol
(D) administration of exogenous androgens
(E) combination chemotherapy

399. A 12-year-old boy, previously in perfect health, suffers a traumatic rupture of the spleen in an automobile accident. He undergoes an emergency splenectomy. All the following sequelae would be expected EXCEPT for

(A) normal splenic function one year later
(B) the appearance of intracellular Heinz bodies in the peripheral blood
(C) a white blood cell count of $20{,}000/mm^3$
(D) overwhelming infection with *Hemophilus influenzae*
(E) a temporary requirement for anticoagulant therapy

400. Aplastic anemia, a condition in which an acellular or markedly hypocellular bone marrow results in pancytopenia, may be caused by all the following EXCEPT

(A) systemic lupus erythematosus
(B) infectious hepatitis
(C) paroxysmal cold hemoglobinuria
(D) paroxysmal nocturnal hemoglobinuria
(E) pregnancy

DIRECTIONS: Each question below contains four suggested answers of which **one** or **more** is correct. Choose the answer:

A	if	**1, 2, and 3**	are correct
B	if	**1 and 3**	are correct
C	if	**2 and 4**	are correct
D	if	**4**	is correct
E	if	**1, 2, 3, and 4**	are correct

401. Sickle-cell anemia is the most prevalent form of congenital hemolytic anemia. Correct statements about this disease include which of the following?

(1) Because of reduced splenic function, affected patients tend to have frequent and severe bacterial infections, especially with gram-negative organisms
(2) Daily supplements of folic acid help in the management of the anemia associated with sickle-cell disease
(3) Splenectomy is advisable after the first **painful** crisis
(4) Most affected patients have isosthenuria and are unable to concentrate their urine

402. Treated polycythemia vera is unlikely to be fatal in less than 12 years. Over this period of time, accepted therapies for this disease include which of the following?

(1) Administration of allopurinol
(2) Administration of cyproheptadine
(3) Administration of chlorambucil
(4) Transfusion of red blood cells

403. A 30-year-old woman with chronic idiopathic thrombocytopenic purpura is admitted to a hospital for management of her second episode of gastrointestinal bleeding. Her only treatment had been 10 mg of prednisone daily for the past six months. Purpura is obvious over her upper chest and neck. Her spleen is palpable one cm below the left costal margin. Platelet count is 10,000/mm^3. Her sedimentation rate is normal and there is no fever. Correct statements about this patient include which of the following?

(1) Splenectomy should be performed after an increased dose of steroids has increased the platelet count
(2) A palpable spleen is an unusual finding
(3) Pregnancy could result in a child born with transient thrombocytopenic purpura
(4) If splenectomy fails, azathioprine is likely to reduce thrombocytopenia

SUMMARY OF DIRECTIONS

A	B	C	D	E
1, 2, 3 only	1, 3 only	2, 4 only	4 only	All are correct

404. A 70-year-old man is brought to an emergency room with gross hematuria and symptoms and signs of hypovolemic shock. Physical examination allows the almost certain diagnosis of cancer of the prostate. He is found to have thrombocytopenia (49,000 platelets/mm^3) and elevated levels of fibrinopeptide A and fibrinogen degradation products. This patient is likely to benefit from which of the following therapies?

(1) The immediate transfusion of whole blood
(2) Large doses of heparin
(3) The administration of estrogens
(4) The administration of fibrinogen and fresh platelets

405. A 40-year-old woman who has metastatic breast cancer is being treated with a combination of cyclophosphamide, vincristine, prednisone, methotrexate, and 5-fluorouracil. Her physician notes that she is troubled with constipation, nocturia, and polyuria. The differential diagnosis includes which of the following?

(1) Steroid-induced diabetes mellitus
(2) Hypercalcemia
(3) Vincristine toxicity
(4) Cyclophosphamide-induced cystitis

406. Of the many causes of hypochromic microcytic anemia, iron deficiency is by far the most common. In diagnosing true iron deficiency anemia, it is correct to say that

(1) absence of detectable iron stored in the marrow occurs early in the development of iron deficiency
(2) mean corpuscular hemoglobin concentration will fall before mean corpuscular volume
(3) measurement of serum ferritin provides a reliable estimate of iron storage and may remove the necessity for bone marrow examination
(4) successful iron replacement can be monitored by the reticulocyte response, which should increase within three days of commencing therapy

407. A 20-year-old man is being investigated for severe normocytic normochromic anemia (hematocrit 28%). Mild granulocytopenia and thrombocytopenia are present. The patient is found to have hemosiderinuria but no hemoglobinuria. He has a low leukocyte alkaline phosphatase level and low red blood cell acetylcholinesterase level. Management of this condition should include

(1) corticosteroid treatment
(2) whole blood transfusions
(3) administration of heparin
(4) administration of fluoxymesterone, 20-30 mg/day

408. Hemophilia is a genetically transmitted bleeding disorder (sex linked recessive pattern) characterized by a deficiency in the procoagulant activities of factor VIII. Correct statements about this condition include which of the following?

(1) Males with the disorder transmit the gene to all their daughters, and neither daughters nor sons will have a bleeding tendency
(2) Fifty percent of female carriers can be detected at a 95 percent confidence level
(3) In 30 percent of cases no family history can be elicited
(4) Hemophilia has an incidence of 1 in 100,000 of the population

409. Hypercalcemia, a common complication of malignancy, can be effectively treated by which of the following measures?

(1) Saline hydration and furosemide administration
(2) Prednisone administration
(3) Mithramycin administration
(4) Calcitonin administration

DIRECTIONS: The groups of questions below consist of lettered choices followed by several numbered items. For each numbered item select the **one** lettered choice with which it is **most** closely associated. Each lettered choice may be used once, more than once, or not at all.

Questions 410-414

Match the following.

(A) Hodgkin's disease
(B) Non-Hodgkin's lymphoma
(C) Both
(D) Neither

410. The age incidence in the United States has a bimodal distribution with one peak between the ages of 15 and 34 years and the other after the age of 50

411. The nodular pattern of the various histologic types has a better prognosis than the diffuse pattern

412. Affected patients are benefited by irradiation, alkylating agents, vinca alkaloids, adriamycin, and bleomycin

413. Symptoms of pruritus and alcohol-induced pain put affected patients in the "B" category and indicate a worse prognosis than if these symptoms were absent

414. The variants of this class of malignant disease are uniformly fatal

Questions 415-419

Match the following.

(A) Acute lymphocytic leukemia
(B) Acute myelocytic leukemia
(C) Both
(D) Neither

415. Disease occurs most frequently in children and may be curable

416. If the affected patient is untreated or fails to respond to therapy, disease is usually fatal within three months, although in individual cases the course of disease can be quite variable

417. Histochemical tests are useful in determining morphologic subtypes. Affected cells usually stain positively with peroxidase and Sudan black stain and are negative for para-aminosalicylic acid stain

418. Chromosomal abnormalities occur and are diagnostic

419. Treatment requires a strategy of intensive chemotherapy that renders affected patients severely hypoplastic or aplastic for a period of time, calling for intensive supportive care measures

Questions 420-424

Match the following.

(A) Myasthenia gravis
(B) Myasthenic syndrome (Eaton-Lambert syndrome)
(C) Both
(D) Neither

420. Associated with thymoma

421. Associated with small cell carcinoma of the lung

422. The physiologic defect is at the neuromuscular junction

423. Affected patients may respond to neostigmine

424. Affected patients may respond to guanidine hydrochloride

Questions 425-429

Match the following.

(A) Benign gastric ulcer
(B) Malignant gastric ulcer
(C) Both
(D) Neither

425. Affected patients may present with epigastric distress, easy fatigability, anemia, and guaiac-positive stools

426. Affected patients respond to antacid therapy both symptomatically and roentgenographically

427. Affected patients may be genetically predisposed to this disease

428. Differential diagnosis includes lymphoma, pseudolymphoma, and Menetrier's disease

429. Disease may be associated with elevated carcinoembryonic antigen titers

Questions 430-434

Match the following.

(A) Methotrexate
(B) Cytosine arabinoside
(C) Nitrogen mustard
(D) Cyclophosphamide
(E) Adriamycin

430. A synthetic alkylating agent that must be activated by the mixed function oxidases in hepatic microsomes. Hydration and adequate urinary flow help to prevent cystitis resulting from this drug

431. A synthetic alkylating agent that, being very reactive in aqueous solution, must be used within minutes of solubilization. May cause a severe chemical burn (cellulitis) if, when injected intravenously, it extravasates into subcutaneous tissues

432. A folic acid antagonist that is excreted by the kidneys essentially unchanged. Renal function must be assessed, therefore, prior to use. Chronic use may produce hepatic cirrhosis

433. A pyrimidine antagonist that functions as a DNA polymerase inhibitor. Major use is in treatment of acute nonlymphocytic leukemia

434. An antitumor antibiotic that is very useful in the treatment of the lymphomas, sarcomas, acute leukemia, and breast cancer. Chronic use may produce fatal cardiomyopathy

Questions 435-439

Match the following.

(A) Vincristine
(B) Vinblastine
(C) Bleomycin
(D) Prednisone
(E) Lomustine (CCNU)

435. An antibiotic, isolated from *Streptomyces verticillus,* effective in treating lymphomas and squamous cell neoplasms. While it has minimal bone marrow toxicity, its use is limited by pulmonary toxicity

436. A plant alkaloid useful in the treatment of leukemias and lymphomas. While it has no bone marrow toxicity, its use is limited by neurotoxicity predominantly affecting the peripheral nervous system

437. A plant alkaloid useful in the treatment of lymphomas, testicular cancer, and breast cancer. Its major dose-limiting toxicity is bone marrow suppression

438. Its main mechanism of action is through alkylation of DNA. Its dose-limiting factor is bone marrow toxicity that may not be evident until three to four weeks after it is administered. Useful in the treatment of lymphomas and brain tumors

439. It lacks bone marrow-suppressant effects. Useful in the treatment of acute lymphocytic leukemia, lymphomas, and breast cancer. Its toxicity is manifested through sodium retention, gastric hyperacidity, hypertension, and glucose intolerance

Questions 440-444

Match the following.

(A) 6-Mercaptopurine (Purinethol)
(B) 5-Fluorouracil
(C) Busulfan (Myeleran)
(D) Chlorambucil (Leukeran)
(E) Leucovorin (citrovorum factor)

440. A synthetic alkylating agent useful in the treatment of chronic myelocytic leukemia. Its long-term use may affect skin pigmentation or cause pulmonary fibrosis

441. A reduced form of folic acid. An antidote to methotrexate toxicity

442. When converted to the ribonucleotide form, inhibits thymidylate synthetase. Useful in the treatment of breast cancer and gastrointestinal neoplasms

443. A synthetic alkylating agent useful in the treatment of chronic lymphocytic leukemia and lymphocytic lymphomas

444. Is converted to its active ribonucleotide form by the enzyme hypoxanthine-guanine phosphoribosyl transferase (HGPRT). Useful in the treatment of acute leukemias, its dose-limiting toxicity is bone marrow suppression

Questions 445-449

Match the following.

(A) Squamous cell (epidermoid) carcinoma
(B) Small cell carcinoma
(C) Adenocarcinoma
(D) Large cell carcinoma
(E) None of the above

445. The most common form of primary lung cancer

446. May cause superior vena caval obstruction, as well as hypercalcemia from ectopic secretion of parathormone-like material

447. Associated with "scar" cancer

448. Associated with a variety of ectopic hormone paraneoplastic syndromes

449. Usually disseminated at the time of diagnosis and the five-year survival rate, despite therapy, is negligible

Oncology and Hematology

Answers

396. The answer is C. *(Isselbacher, ed 9. pp 1637-1639.)* The Ann Arbor staging classification of the lymphomas is as follows:

Stage I: Involvement of one lymph node region only (I) or of a single extralymphatic organ or site (I_E).

Stage II: Involvement of two or more lymph node regions on the same side of the diaphragm either alone (II) or involving a contiguous extralymphatic organ or tissue (II_E).

Stage III: Involvement of lymph node regions on both sides of the diaphragm (III), which may also include the spleen (III_S), contiguous extralymphatic organs (III_E), or both (III_{ES}).

Stage IV: Multiple or disseminated foci of involvement of one or more extralymphatic organs or tissues, with or without lymphatic involvement.

Accordingly, the patient presented in the question will have stage III_E because of disease above and below the diaphragm, as well as involvement of the pulmonary parenchyma which is contiguous to the hilar lymph node region. Should this patient have had discrete pulmonary parenchymal lesions, the clinical stage would have been IV. In addition, the presence of fever and weight loss of more than 10 percent are the cardinal symptoms of Hodgkin's disease and are designated as "B" in the staging system. The absence of these symptoms is designated as "A."

397. The answer is E. *(Isselbacher, ed 9. pp 1523-1524.)* Vitamin B_{12} deficiency occurs in 100 percent of patients following total gastrectomy; after partial gastrectomy, vitamin B_{12} deficiency is variable. Such deficiencies, which frequently are owing to intestinal overgrowth of bacteria, may respond to antibiotics. A classical hematological finding in megaloblastic anemia is an MCV greater than 96 μm^3; frequently, the MCV exceeds 110 μm^3. The reticulocyte count is low and leukocyte and platelet counts may be diminished, especially in the presence of severe anemia. Megaloblastic anemia is further distinguished by pronounced anicytosis and poikilocytosis and by the presence of macroovalocytes; basophilic stippling and an occasional nucleated red blood cell are also seen, and neutropenia is common. Enhanced intramedullary destruction of erythroblasts results in an increase in the plasma level of lactic acid dehydrogenase. Vitamin B_{12} plasma levels usually fall to below 100 pg/ml before clinically significant disease develops.

398. The answer is E. *(Holland, pp 1769-1787. Isselbacher, ed 9. pp 1792-1794.)* The history presented in the question offers two very unfavorable prognostic features for the woman involved: first, the shortness of the disease-free interval, i.e., one year following her mastectomy; and second, the appearance of visceral metastases as the first indication of recurrence of cancer. These are also signs of a very aggressive disease process. Had this patient presented with soft tissue metastases, e.g., in skin or regional nodes, she might have been a candidate for hormonal manipulation if a tumor specimen furnished evidence of estrogen and progesterone receptors. A favorable response to hormonal manipulation occurs in approximately 50 to 75 percent of receptor-positive patients. In contrast, the response to hormonal manipulation is only 10 percent in receptor-negative patients. In women who have visceral metastases, the response to hormonal manipulation not only is poorer, but several months must pass before objective evidence of a response appears. Quicker responses with combination chemotherapy, e.g., cyclophosphamide, methotrexate, and 5-fluorouracil, are available for such patients; such would be the treatment of choice for this woman.

399. The answer is D. *(Isselbacher, ed 9. p 1581.)* Removal of a spleen that has been damaged by traumatic rupture is a common surgical procedure; thus, significant data exist concerning the effects of this operation on host defense mechanisms. Of the numerous sequelae that follow, an increase in susceptibility to infection following removal of the spleen in patients with diseases of that organ is not a common one. Thus, it would be surprising to have an otherwise healthy child overcome by *Haemophilus influenzae* infection. The hematological changes associated with removal of all splenic function, mainly the appearance of red blood cells with Howell-Jolly bodies, acanthocytes and siderocytes, Heinz bodies, and target cells all would be expected. Normal splenic function may be found in patients within a year of splenectomy. In many instances this restoration of function will be due to the presence of an accessory spleen that has appropriately hypertrophied; recent evidence, however, would suggest that, in the vast majority of children who undergo splenectomy, rudimentary splenic tissue present in all individuals expands into a functioning organ. Within two weeks of surgery, a leukocytosis of 20,000/mm^3 and a thrombocytosis exceeding 1,000,000/mm^3 are not uncommon. Because a steep rise in platelet count can be associated with portal vein thrombosis, prophylactic anticoagulant therapy should be instituted if the platelet level approaches this figure.

400. The answer is C. *(Isselbacher, ed 9. pp 1525-1526.)* Failure of stem cell differentiation in the bone marrow results in pancytopenia, which involves a lack of erythrocytes, neutrophils, and platelets. The term aplastic anemia should be restricted to states involving this degree of hypocellularity. A few patients appear to develop aplastic anemia because of immunological mechanisms that lead to the destruction of bone marrow stem cells or prevent their normal maturation. Such mechanisms may be operative in the infrequent, but well-described, aplastic anemia associated with active systemic lupus erythematosus. It is of interest that immunoregulatory T cells, which are disordered in this condition, have also been demonstrated to be capable of influencing erythroid precursor-cell maturation. Both infectious hepatitis (A) and serum hepatitis (B) may be associated with the development of aplastic anemia, a complication that is not necessarily related to the severity of the hepatitis and that usually develops as the hepatitis is resolving. Aplastic anemia is an extremely dangerous complication of hepatitis; in many affected patients the bone marrow suppression is reported to be profound and irreversible. Aplastic anemia can develop in the course of paroxysmal nocturnal hemoglobinuria and as a complication of pregnancy. In the latter condition, the bone marrow suppression may remit following delivery of the fetus. Paroxysmal cold hemoglobinuria today is a rare disorder; formerly, it occurred in association with tertiary syphilis as a result of the formation of an IgG antibody directed against the P antigen on the surface of red blood cells. Now that syphilis has again become prevalent, paroxysmal cold hemoglobinuria also may reappear with increasing frequency. Rarely, idiopathic cases of paroxysmal cold hemoglobinuria may occur, but such cases have not been associated with the development of an aplastic anemia.

401. The answer is D (4). *(Isselbacher, ed 9. p 1547.)* The differential diagnosis of hemolytic anemia in black patients includes sickle cell disease. A positive sickling test will indicate a genetic abnormality that results in the production of an abnormal hemoglobin. The hemoglobin forms, which represent the phenotypic expression of these genetic abnormalities, are not necessarily associated with disease. To diagnose sickle cell anemia, with its characteristic SS phenotype, hemoglobin electrophoresis is needed inasmuch as subjects with an AS phenotype and double heterozygotes also will manifest abnormal sickling. The spleen plays a vital role in defense against bacterial infection. It is a major lymphoid organ capable of rapidly producing antibodies—especially IgM. It also has a major reticuloendothelial function that is important in the clearing of opsonized and phagocytosed bacteria. Because these functions are impaired in patients with sickle cell disease, frequent and severe bacterial infections result. Pneumococcal organisms and other polysaccharide-containing antigens provide the most severe problems for these patients. Splenectomy will help neither their sickling tendencies nor their host defense mechanisms, but may provide symptomatic relief from the painful crises that are associated with the engorgement of the reticuloendothelial system of the spleen.

402. The answer is E (all). *(Isselbacher, ed 9. pp 1576-1579.)* Polycythemia vera, so named to distinguish it from the physiological polycythemia that can follow anoxia, is one of the myeloproliferative syndromes. For diagnosis of polycythemia vera, demonstration of a marked increase in total red blood cell mass accompanied by an elevated hemoglobin concentration is necessary. Repeated phlebotomy will lower the red blood cell mass. This procedure is often combined with busulfan or chlorambucil administration to suppress the rate of maturation of erythroid precursors. As is the case in patients with psoriasis, the massive cell turnover in polycythemia vera, especially after treatment with cytotoxic agents, will lead to the release of large amounts of uric acid that may precipitate a gouty arthritis. Prophylactic use of allopurinol in doses of 300 mg/day is recommended to prevent this complication. Patients with polycythemia vera often have a severe pruritus that frequently responds to cyproheptadine in a dose of 12-16 mg/day. The natural history of this disease frequently involves a leukemic phase that may prove fatal. Fifteen to 20 percent of affected patients who do not develop leukemia undergo marrow fibrosis, splenomegaly, and serious anemia.

403. The answer is E (all). *(Isselbacher, ed 9. pp 1556-1557.)* Idiopathic thrombocytopenic purpura (ITP), a disease that perhaps is more accurately referred to as autoimmune thrombocytopenic purpura, has both an acute and chronic form. The acute form occurs more frequently in children than adults, whereas the chronic recurrent form predominates in women who are in the second to fourth decade of life. The disease is characterized by transient remissions and exacerbations that can last for weeks or months, and in some cases years. A palpable spleen is unusual in ITP; splenomegaly, even in the 10 percent of patients who have it, usually is minimal. Although splenectomy does not cure the underlying disease process, it does remove the organ in which damaged platelets are destroyed. Splenectomy is indicated in patients who have failed to recover spontaneously within three-to-six months of the onset of their illness and in those patients who require more than 10 mg of prednisone per day for three months. ITP almost certainly is due to the presence of antiplatelet antibodies, which can be detected in at least 80 percent of affected patients. However, demonstration of these antibodies is made difficult by their inability to fix complement. Platelet antibodies have been demonstrated by measuring (1) an increased secretion of platelet factor 3 caused by exposure of normal platelets to IgG fractions from the serum of patients with ITP, (2) the release of platelet serotonin by platelets exposed to serum of affected patients, and (3) the stimulation of lymphocytes from patients with ITP by serum-platelet complexes from affected patients. Beginning with the 18th week of fetal life, the IgG antibody that produces ITP can readily cross the placenta; thus, infants of mothers affected with this disease are frequently born with a transient ITP. In patients who do not respond to splenectomy, drug treatment with vincristine, cyclophosphamide, or azathioprine frequently is helpful by increasing platelet survival in 50-70 percent of such cases. However, this initially favorable response to therapy usually is not sustained. Generally, in such situations vincristine is the drug of choice because it has the least effect on bone marrow.

404. The answer is B (1, 3). *(Isselbacher, ed 9. p 1566.)* Numerous metabolic and physical stimuli may produce the profound hypofibrinogenemia associated with the consumption of fibrinogen by intravascular clotting. This syndrome, known as disseminated intravascular coagulation (DIC), may be produced by (1) snake bites, (2) hypovolemic shock, (3) anaphylaxis, (4) bacterial septicemia, and (5) various neoplasms, particularly carcinoma of the prostate. Despite the tendency of patients with this complication to hemorrhage, it is necessary to treat them with anticoagulants to prevent further intravascular clotting. Heparin, although effective, if administered alone may increase the risk of hemorrhage; therefore, it is usually given with fresh plasma to replace the fibrinogen that is being absorbed. The use of plasma alone would simply supply more fibrinogen to act as a substrate for clotting enzymes. If bleeding is severe, whole blood will be required. Platelet transfusion may be necessary if thrombocytopenia is significant. Smaller doses of heparin are administered in the face of severe thrombocytopenia. Apart from these emergency measures, the long-term treatment for DIC is directed at the underlying disease process. If a carcinoma of the prostate is sensitive to estrogen therapy, estrogen administration will rapidly reverse DIC. Acute leukemia and lymphomas, as well as solid neoplasms involving the pancreas and bronchial tree, also are frequently associated with DIC.

405. The answer is A (1, 2, 3). *(Holland, p 1079. Isselbacher, ed 9. p 1735.)* The polyuria and nocturia in the patient discussed in the question may well be secondary to steroid-induced diabetes mellitus. Vincristine is a neurotoxin. While it predominantly affects the peripheral nervous system as manifested in a loss of deep tendon reflexes, an early sign of vincristine neurotoxicity is constipation. Therefore, patients receiving this drug should pay close attention to bowel movements and perhaps take stool softeners and bulk laxatives temporarily. With its strong propensity for producing osteolytic metastases, breast cancer is a common cause of hypercalcemia. Among the earliest symptoms of hypercalcemia are nocturia and polyuria resulting from the inhibitory effect of calcium on antidiuretic hormone action on the distal tubule. Hypercalcemia also inhibits smooth muscle contractility, causing constipation. Cyclophosphamide-induced cystitis promotes urgency and frequency with the voiding of small amounts of urine, not polyuria.

406. The answer is B (1, 3). *(Isselbacher, ed 9. pp 1516-1517.)* Patients with chronic conditions such as rheumatoid arthritis often have a low serum iron level, whereas their total iron stores, as seen in a marrow biopsy, are within normal limits. In genuinely iron-deficient patients, no stainable iron will be present in marrow tissue. As total iron body stores fall, corpuscular volume decreases and, in a more chronic stage, mean corpuscular hemoglobin concentration falls. The need for pursuing bone marrow tissue has been reduced by the finding that serum ferritin levels correlate extremely well with tissue stores of iron. In severe cases of iron deficiency anemia, serum ferritin levels may fall by as much as 90 percent. In such cases, free erythrocyte porphyrin is usually elevated. The mainstay of therapy for iron deficiency anemia continues to be ferrous sulfate. It is important to follow the progress of the therapy during the first ten days with serial reticulocyte counts. Reticulocytosis can be expected after the seventh, and before the tenth, day of replacement therapy with ferrous sulfate.

407. The answer is C (2, 4). *(Isselbacher, ed 9. pp 1540-1541.)* The patient presented in the question almost certainly suffers from paroxysmal nocturnal hemoglobinuria (PNH). Notwithstanding the name of the syndrome, hemoglobinuria is seldom gross and may occur only intermittently—in some affected patients no more than trace amounts may ever occur. Similarly, the anemia associated with this condition is variable, being profound in only a few patients. Most patients exhibit normal levels of hemoglobin or only moderate reductions. The diagnosis, however, would be extremely unlikely in the absence of hemosiderin in the urine. A preliminary diagnosis of PNH is confirmed with an acid hemolysis test or sucrose lysis test. Further confirmation would be evidence of low concentrations of leukocyte alkaline phosphatase and red blood cell acetylcholinesterase. Activation of the terminal part of the complement cascade normally is associated with some red blood cell lysis. However, patients with PNH are inordinately sensitive to these complement components. In addition to erythrocytes, granulocytes and platelets also are sensitive to these mechanisms. Transfusions of whole blood are usually beneficial. Although blood transfusions will contain some complement components and their substrates, this potential danger is offset by the passive increase in hemoglobin levels that follows transfusion. The increase in hemoglobin will suppress bone marrow production of young erythrocytes, which are particularly sensitive to complement. For similar reasons, the administration of ferrous sulfate to promote increased erythropoiesis will lead to the production of excessive numbers of young erythrocytes that will be destroyed by complement. Therapy with androgens, such as fluoxymesterone, frequently decreases the destruction of red blood cells and allows hemoglobin levels to rise. These steroids have been shown to affect both complement and red blood cells; however, their mechanism of action in this disease is not certain. PNH frequently is complicated by venous thromboses, for which prophylactic anticoagulation will be necessary. Coumarin type drugs are useful in such situations, but heparin, which has been found actually to increase the rate of hemolysis, should be avoided.

408. The answer is A (1, 2, 3). *(Isselbacher, ed 9. pp 1560-1561.)* With the improved treatment for hemophilia, it is theoretically possible that a growing number of affected males could pass the abnormal gene on to their progeny. Inasmuch as sex (or the lack of femaleness) is determined by the male Y chromosome, all sons of men with hemophilia will be normal. However, all daughters of such patients will possess the abnormal gene. Thus, the major emphasis continues to be placed on the detection of female carriers. Hemophilia follows the sex-linked inheritance pattern. Mothers may expect 50 percent of their sons to be affected by the disease and 50 percent of their daughters to carry the abnormal gene. Fortunately, it is now possible with a high degree of accuracy to detect female carriers. The test involves the determination of both the antigenicity of factor VIII in suspected carriers as well as the serum level of functional factor VIII. By examining both properties of factor VIII, 30 percent of carriers can be detected at the 99 percent level of confidence and at least 50 percent at the 95 percent confidence level. Spontaneous mutations on the X chromosome obviously occur, for as many as 30 percent of hemophiliac individuals have no family history of the disease. Of the inherited disturbances in coagulation, hemophilia is the most common—it affects one in every 10,000 births.

409. The answer is E (all). *(Holland, pp 1081-1082. Isselbacher, ed 9. p 1837.)* A variety of measures are effective for the treatment of hypercalcemia secondary to neoplasms. Minimally elevated serum calcium, i.e., in the 11 to 12 mg/100 ml range, will respond to simple saline hydration and diuresis. Higher serum calcium levels may warrant the addition of other agents such as prednisone. This drug is most effective in treating the hypercalcemia caused by tumors, against which it exerts effective oncolytic action. Mithramycin diminishes serum calcium levels through its inhibition of osteoclastic activity. Calcitonin, the physiologic antagonist of parathyroid hormone, reduces bone resorption and increases the renal clearance of calcium.

410-414. The answers are: 410-A, 411-B, 412-C, 413-D, 414-D. *(Isselbacher, ed 9. pp 1635, 1641-1646, 1651.)* Whereas Hodgkin's disease has a bimodal distribution of age incidence in the United States, with a peak between the ages of 15 and 35 and another after 50, non-Hodgkin's lymphomas have a single peak, occurring chiefly after the age of 50. The major histologic subtypes of Hodgkin's disease are nodular sclerosis, mixed cellularity, lymphocyte predominance, and lymphocyte depletion. The best prognosis is associated with the nodular sclerosing and lymphocyte-predominant varieties. While the histologic picture can be very pleomorphic, the malignant cell in Hodgkin's disease is believed to be the Reed-Sternberg cell, a dedifferentiated histiocyte.

It is important to distinguish the non-Hodgkin's lymphomas by histologic pattern as well as cell type, because the prognosis is better with the nodular pattern than with the diffuse. The Rappaport classification is currently used for the non-Hodgkin's lymphomas, which include lymphocytic poorly differentiated, lymphocytic well differentiated, histiocytic, and mixed lymphocytic-histiocytic. The well differentiated lymphocytic lymphomas have the best overall prognosis and at times are difficult to distinguish from chronic lymphocytic leukemia. Nodal presentation is associated with 90 percent of patients who have Hodgkin's disease; in the non-Hodgkin's lymphomas, extranodal presentation is much more common.

The "B" symptoms carrying major prognostic significance in Hodgkin's disease are fever, night sweats, and unexplained weight loss exceeding 10 percent of the total body weight. While pruritus and alcohol-induced pain may be symptoms of the lymphomas, chiefly Hodgkin's disease, their presence does not indicate a poorer prognosis. There is a question as to whether "B" symptoms have an important prognostic significance in the non-Hodgkin's lymphomas.

All lymphomas can benefit from the treatments listed in question 412; the optimum combination of drugs or irradiation, or both, can cure 25 to 90 percent of patients afflicted with Hodgkin's disease and 50 percent of patients who have non-Hodgkin's lymphomas, depending on their histologic subtype.

The treatment of choice for stage I and II Hodgkin's disease is irradiation; stages III and IV are usually treated with various combinations of drugs together with irradiation. The drug combination most commonly used is known as MOPP, consisting of mechlorethamine (Mustargen), vincristine (Oncovin), prednisone, and procarbazine. Localized (stage I) non-Hodgkin's lymphoma is optimally treated with local irradiation; various drug combinations are used to treat the more advanced stages of the disease.

415-419. The answers are: 415-A, 416-C, 417-B, 418-C, 419-B. *(Isselbacher, ed 9. pp 1621-1629, 1632-1633.)* The peak incidence of acute lymphocytic leukemia (ALL) is between the ages of two and four years. Although the disease also occurs in adults, adult leukemia is predominantly myelogenous (myelocytic, myelomonocytic, monocytic promyelocytic, and erythroleukemia). The sexes are equally affected in very young children; however, in older patients, ALL shows a slight male predominance (3:2).

All acute leukemia patients who fail to respond to therapy have a median survival of approximately three months. Death usually results from one of the complications of bone marrow failure, i.e., infection or bleeding or both. However, modern therapy allows 90 to 95 percent of children who have ALL to enter remission; the median survival is approximately five years. It is projected that 25 percent of these patients may be cured. Acute leukemia therapy is divided into several stages: induction, consolidation, central nervous system prophylaxis, and maintenance. Although approximately 50 percent of patients who have acute myelocytic leukemia (AML) will enter complete remission, the median duration of their remissions is only 10 to 12 months owing to a lack of effective measures to maintain the remission.

It is important to distinguish the two major forms of acute leukemia because the choice of therapy and prognosis in each is quite different. This differentiation can frequently be accomplished by the examination of Wright-stained smears of the bone marrow. In ALL, the lymphoblasts have a high nuclear:cytoplasmic ratio, scant nucleoli (one or two), no Auer rods, and the myeloid elements that are present appear normal. The lymphoblasts stain positively with para-aminosalicylic acid (PAS) and negatively with peroxidase and Sudan black. In contrast, leukemic myeloblasts contain more nucleoli (two to four) in a homogenous "ground glass" nucleus. Auer rods may be evident in the cytoplasm and other more mature myeloid elements may be abnormal. The myeloblasts stain positively with peroxidase and Sudan black and negatively with PAS.

Chromosomal abnormalities may be quite common in the blasts of acute leukemia. Fifty percent of patients who have AML exhibit some chromosomal abnormality in number or structure or both, using standard techniques: these abnormalities vary from patient to patient. With improved techniques, however, according to a recent report, such abnormalities may be far more common than was formerly believed. The only leukemia with a fairly consistent chromosomal abnormality is chronic myelocytic leukemia, in which 90 percent of affected patients have the Philadelphia chromosome.

The four most active drugs for inducing remission in AML are cytosine arabinoside, 6-thioguanine, daunorubicin, and adriamycin, usually given in combination. Each of these drugs destroys normal stem cells of the bone marrow. Consequently, the anemia, granulocytopenia, and thrombocytopenia that testify to the myelophthisic effects of the disease are severely aggravated by the indiscriminate effects of these drugs. Therefore, during chemotherapy, patients who have AML must receive meticulous supportive care with blood products and antibiotics if the consequences of bone marrow failure are to be ameliorated. In contrast, prednisone, vincristine, and asparaginase, the drugs most capable of inducing remission in children who have ALL, do not destroy the normal myeloid elements of bone marrow.

420-424. The answers are: 420-A, 421-B, 422-C, 423-A, 424-B. *(Isselbacher, ed 9. pp 2066-2067.)* Both myasthenia gravis and the myasthenic syndrome (Eaton-Lambert syndrome) may be associated with tumors—the former with lymphoblastic and epithelial tumors of the thymus, the latter with small cell carcinoma of the lung. Since the myasthenic syndrome may precede the appearance of the tumor by as much as two years, and because response to therapy may be quite different for the two myasthenic disorders, they must be carefully distinguished.

Both conditions involve abnormalities at the myoneural junction. However, the conditions can be differentiated on an anatomic, physiologic, and pharmacologic basis, as well as by their association with other morbid conditions. Although myasthenia gravis generally occurs independently of other disorders, 8 to 10 percent of myasthenic patients have a tumor of the thymus gland. Removal of this tumor may result in improvement of the myasthenia gravis. The muscle groups characteristically affected in myasthenia gravis are the facial, oculomotor, laryngeal, pharyngeal, and respiratory. Late in the disease, the shoulder and pelvic muscles also become involved. In contrast, the myasthenic syndrome, which usually spares the bulbar musculature, initially weakens the muscles of the pelvic and shoulder girdles. Each disorder has characteristic electromyographic findings. Myasthenia gravis exhibits a characteristic "myasthenic fatigability" pattern evoked by rapid repetitive stimuli. In the myasthenic syndrome, however, electromyography reveals a recruitment phenomenon involving an initially low amplitude pattern that, with rapid repetitive stimuli, increases.

The edrophonium chloride (Tensilon) test is also helpful in distinguishing myasthenia gravis from the myasthenic syndrome. Tensilon is the preferred cholinesterase antagonist for diagnostic purposes because the response to it is nearly instantaneous and its effect vanishes in minutes. In true myasthenia gravis, Tensilon causes dramatic improvement in muscle strength. Affected patients who so respond to Tensilon can be treated safely with longer-acting cholinesterase inhibitors, such as neostigmine. While cholinesterase inhibitors have little or no effect on the muscle weakness of the myasthenic syndrome, muscle function in this disorder can be dramatically restored either by removing the associated tumor or controlling it with irradiation or chemotherapy, or both. If neither is possible, palliative therapy with guanidine hydrochloride may improve muscle strength. Both groups of affected patients are inordinately sensitive to small doses of tubocurarine and decamethonium.

425-429. The answers are: 425-C, 426-C, 427-B, 428-B, 429-B. *(Isselbacher, ed 9. pp 1378-1379, 1385-1386.)* The clinical histories associated with benign and malignant gastric ulcers tend to be quite similar. The peak incidence for benign ulcer disease is between 45 and 55 years of age; for gastric carcinoma, it is 55 years of age. Both benign and malignant ulcer diseases affect men more frequently than women, the ratio being 3.5:1 for the benign disease, and 2:1 for the malignant. While benign gastric ulcer disease does not appear to have a familial predisposition, gastric cancer is two to four times more common in relatives of affected patients than in the general population.

Symptoms of benign gastric ulcers may be quite vague; easy satiety and nausea after eating are common complaints. Midepigastric pain may be aggravated by eating, and weight loss is frequent. Bleeding results in guaiac-positive stools, and secondary anemia and weight loss result in easy fatigability.

Although the clinical history associated with benign gastric ulcers is shared by the majority of patients afflicted with malignant gastric ulcers, approximately 25 percent of such patients present classic **duodenal** ulcer symptoms, including midepigastric burning pain relieved by food.

Preoperative differentiation between benign and malignant ulcer disease is possible in 80 to 90 percent of cases. Radiology can accurately differentiate between them approximately 85 percent of the time. Gastroscopy, cytologic examination, and biopsy of the lesions yield a diagnostic accuracy as high as 90 percent. False-positive cytologic results are exceeding uncommon, most diagnostic errors arising from false-negatives. Examination of gastric acid is very helpful; true achlorhydria following maximal pentagastrin stimulation almost always excludes a benign gastric ulcer. Yet the presence of acid does not rule out gastric carcinoma. Moreover, improvement in response to medical therapy, both subjectively and on x-ray, can occur in patients who have malignant ulcers. If, following testing, doubt persists as to whether or not the lesion is benign, the affected patient should have surgery.

Conditions that often mimic malignant ulcers on x-ray include peptic ulcer disease, hypertrophic pyloric stenosis, antral gastritis, inflammatory polyps, Menetrier's disease, lymphoma, pseudolymphoma, Crohn's disease, gastric varices, hematoma, and bezoars or retained food. Unfortunately, carcinoembryonic antigen titers reach diagnostic levels only after cancer has metastasized and, thus, are valueless in early diagnosis.

430-434. The answers are: 430-D, 431-C, 432-A, 433-B, 434-E. *(Holland, pp 739-754, 781-784, 791-806, 826-835. Isselbacher, ed 9. pp 1601-1607.)* Cyclophosphamide in its commercial form is inactive. It was designed in the hope that its chemical activation would be confined to tumor cells. While this is not the case, cyclophosphamide continues to be a very effective antitumor agent. Although the active antitumor metabolites are unidentified, it is certain that they are excreted in the urine. These metabolites are strongly irritating to the bladder mucosa; their effects range from mild dysuria to severe hemorrhagic cystitis and death. Therefore, normal bladder evacuation and a dilute urine are imperative with the use of cyclophosphamide.

Nitrogen mustard was the first chemotherapeutic agent found to be effective against human cancer. Its major use is in the treatment of lymphoproliferative disorders. Toxic manifestations other than those listed in the question include nausea, vomiting, bone marrow suppression, and alopecia.

Methotrexate was synthesized with the deliberate intent to form a potent folate antagonist because of the observation that exogenous folic acid appeared to accelerate the progression of acute leukemia. The drug has a wide tumoricidal spectrum including acute leukemia, breast cancer, head and neck cancer, choriocarcinoma, and osteogenic sarcoma. Major dose-limiting effects of methotrexate include bone marrow suppression and oral and gastrointestinal toxicity.

Cytosine arabinoside (ara-C) is an analog of the naturally occurring cytosine ribonucleoside. It must be activated via cytidine kinase to the active nucleotide AraCTP, which competes with CTP for the polymerase enzyme. Dose-limiting toxicity includes nausea, vomiting, and bone marrow suppression. Because of its short physical half-life this agent must be given in multiple repeated injections or as a constant infusion. Oral ara-C is ineffective because of the high concentration of cytidine deaminase in the intestinal mucosa that converts ara-C to the inactive uracil arabinoside.

Adriamycin is isolated from *Streptomyces peuceteus.* It functions as an inhibitor of DNA synthesis via intercalation into the DNA molecule. Toxicity other than that listed includes nausea, vomiting, bone marrow suppression, alopecia, and stomatitis.

435-439. The answers are: 435-C, 436-A, 437-B, 438-E, 439-D. *(Blum, Cancer 31:903-914, 1973. Holland, pp 840-845. Isselbacher, ed 9. pp 1601-1607.)* Bleomycin inhibits DNA synthesis. The mechanism of inhibition is incompletely understood, but the drug is known to produce double-strand breaks in the DNA molecule. The pulmonary toxicity consists mainly of a diffusion impairment and is a cumulative phenomenon; therefore, patients receiving bleomycin must be monitored with serial pulmonary function tests. Unless there is underlying pulmonary disease, serious pulmonary toxicity is uncommon with total doses under 300 units. Other toxic effects include skin hyperpigmentation and cutaneous ulcers.

Vincristine (Oncovin) is a plant alkaloid that causes a metaphase arrest in both normal and neoplastic cells. Neurotoxic effects are common and consist mainly of loss of deep tendon reflexes, paresthesias in fingers and toes, and constipation. If the drug is continued beyond the point of moderate paresthesias, foot drop and other neurotoxic signs may develop. The neurotoxicity usually subsides within weeks or months after discontinuation of the drug, depending on the severity of the complication.

Vinblastine (Velban) is chemically similar to, and derived from the same source as, vincristine, but differs somewhat in therapeutic spectrum and toxic manifestations. Vinblastine also causes metaphase arrest in normal and neoplastic cells. Like vincristine, it is neurotoxic in large doses, but vinblastine's toxic effect on bone marrow usually precludes doses of a magnitude that would produce neurotoxicity.

Lomustine (CCNU) is one of a new class of alkylating agents known generically as nitrosoureas. These compounds have been shown to be synergistic with other alkylating agents such as cyclophosphamide and with the anthracycline antibiotic, adriamycin.

Prednisone is a synthetic analog of the adrenal glucocorticoids; consequently, its effects on various organs are similar to those observed in Cushing's syndrome or adrenal hyperplasia. The cytolytic action of prednisone is poorly understood, but its lack of bone marrow toxicity makes it an attractive component in drug combinations. Prednisone is also of value in treating the hypercalcemia of malignancy.

440-444. The answers are: 440-C, 441-E, 442-B, 443-D, 444-A. *(Holland, pp 754-760, 774-780, 802-804. Isselbacher, ed 9. pp 1601-1607.)* Busulfan (Myleran) is an alkylating agent administered orally, usually on a daily basis. It is well tolerated, and its major dose-limiting toxicity is bone marrow suppression. In the treatment of chronic myelocytic leukemia, the drug is usually discontinued when the white blood cell count reaches 20,000/mm^3. After cessation of therapy, the count usually falls and may stabilize at approximately 10,000/mm^3. If busulfan is continued inadvertently, it may produce severe and protracted bone marrow hypoplasia.

Leucovorin is frequently used in conjunction with various high-dose methotrexate regimens. Leucovorin is effective either parenterally or orally, and is usually given sequentially following methotrexate. If given concurrently with methotrexate in sufficient dosage, leucovorin will attenuate methotrexate's therapeutic as well as toxic effects.

5-Fluorouracil is inactive in its native form and must be converted to the nucleotide 5-fluorodeoxyuridylate (F-dUMP), in which form it competes with dUMP, the naturally occurring substrate for thymidylate synthetase. By thus inhibiting the biosynthesis of thymidylate, F-dUMP thereby inhibits DNA synthesis. The major dose-limiting toxicity of this drug is bone marrow suppression and oral and gastrointestinal ulceration.

Chlorambucil (Leukeran) is usually given orally on a daily basis and is well tolerated. Its major dose-limiting toxicity is bone marrow suppression.

6-Mercaptopurine (Purinethol) is usually given orally on a daily basis. On rare occasions, it can cause hepatitis. A closely related congener, azathioprine (Imuran), is a popular immunosuppressive agent for the treatment of autoimmune diseases and in the preparation of recipients of kidney transplants. Azathioprine has no distinct advantage over 6-mercaptopurine.

445-449. The answers are: 445-A, 446-A, 447-C, 448-B, 449-B. *(Holland, pp 1473-1518. Isselbacher, ed 9. pp 1260, 1264. Selawry, Semin Oncol 1:163-287, 1974.)* Bronchogenic carcinoma (malignant tumors of the bronchial epithelium) account for 90 percent of all lung malignancies. While not all pathologists agree, the World Health Organization defines four major histologic types: epidermoid (squamous cell), 42 percent; large cell anaplastic, 22 percent; small cell anaplastic, 18 percent; and adenocarcinoma, 10 percent. Bronchogenic carcinoma has reached epidemic proportions throughout the world as a result of environmental pollution and cigarette smoking; all four histologic types have been related to cigarette smoking. The death rates from bronchogenic carcinoma, per 100,000 population, are 3.4 among nonsmokers, 59.3 among smokers of 10 to 20 cigarettes a day, and 217 among smokers of 40 or more cigarettes a day. Other carcinogens that have been implicated include chromates, arsenic, nickel, beryllium, and asbestos.

Squamous cell (epidermoid) carcinoma tends to occur centrally in the tracheobronchial tree. Hence, the symptoms caused by this histologic type often are those of bronchial obstruction, ulceration, or local invasion. Consequently, cough, hemoptysis, hoarseness (due to involvement of the recurrent laryngeal nerve), and signs and symptoms of obstruction of the superior vena cava are frequent. Other bronchogenic histologic types that may produce superior vena caval obstruction include the small and large cell anaplastic variants.

Adenocarcinoma, in contrast to epidermoid carcinoma, generally appears as a peripheral lesion in the apex of the lung and in pre-existing scar tissue, "scar" carcinoma.

While ectopic hormone secretion is most frequently associated with small cell carcinoma of the lung, hypercalcemia due to the elaboration of a parathormone-like hormone is most commonly seen with the epidermoid variant. The ectopic hormones associated with small cell carcinoma usually include antidiuretic and adrenocorticotropic (ACTH) hormones. Patients who have excess ectopic ACTH infrequently show signs of Cushing's disease, however; the clinical clue to ACTH excess is hypokalemic alkalosis. The five-year survival rate for patients afflicted with small cell carcinoma who undergo surgery or irradiation is still less than 5 percent, because at the time of diagnosis the lesion has usually metastasized widely, a development that conventional diagnostic methods fail to detect.

Neurology

DIRECTIONS: Each question below contains five suggested answers. Choose the **one best** response to each question.

450. A 71-year-old man who has been having left-sided headaches and low-grade fever for several weeks suddenly loses vision in his left eye. On admission to a hospital, his erythrocyte sedimentation rate is found to be greatly elevated. Treatment should begin with which of the following drugs?

(A) Heparin
(B) Sulfinpyrazone
(C) Prednisone
(D) Aspirin
(E) Strong analgesics

451. The combination of extensor plantar reflexes and absent ankle reflexes may be due to all the following conditions EXCEPT

(A) vitamin B_{12} deficiency
(B) multiple disc lesions
(C) motor system disease
(D) syringomyelia
(E) tumor of cauda equina

452. An elderly woman is admitted to a hospital in a confused state. Her blood glucose level is 1100 mg/100 ml. The glucose level is brought down promptly to normal by insulin, but the patient's mental state deteriorates, and she becomes semicomatose. Her declining condition is probably attributable to

(A) brain damage produced by the hyperglycemia
(B) cerebral edema and hypo-osmolality caused by the rapid drop in blood glucose
(C) cerebral ischemia due to diabetes and patient's age
(D) onset of lactic acidosis
(E) insulin allergy

453. A young man complains of acute back and right leg pain. On examination he is found to have hypalgesia of the little toes and lateral calf, as well as absence of the ankle reflex, of the right leg. The patient probably has herniation of the disc between which of the following vertebrae?

(A) L2-L3
(B) L3-L4
(C) L4-L5
(D) L5-S1
(E) S1-S2

454. A 54-year-old man complains of one year of intermittent vertigo. On examination, there is hearing loss and absent caloric response of the left ear. Cerebrospinal fluid protein is found to be 110 mg/100 ml. The most likely diagnosis is

(A) labyrinthitis
(B) Meniere's disease
(C) chronic otitis media
(D) acoustic neuroma
(E) vestibular neuronitis

455. A patient arrives at a hospital breathing, but without other evidence of brain function. Two electroencephalograms at 24-hour intervals are both isoelectric. A reasonably good chance of full recovery exists if the underlying factor is

(A) cardiac arrest
(B) intracerebral hemorrhage
(C) encephalitis
(D) head trauma
(E) barbiturate overdose

456. A patient complains of lack of sensitivity and a tingling in the legs and feet, as well as of weakness of the legs. On examination, there is loss of position and vibration sense in the feet, weakness and hyperreflexia of the legs, and bilateral Babinski signs. The lesion responsible for these findings probably involves which of the following regions of the spinal cord?

(A) Lateral
(B) Posterior
(C) Lateral and anterior
(D) Anterior and posterior
(E) Posterior and lateral

457. A 45-year-old man, who is a heavy drinker, is admitted to a hospital with diplopia, mild drowsiness, disorientation, and ataxia of a weeks duration. On examination, this patient is found to be inattentive and cannot concentrate. He is disoriented in time and place, and periodically falls asleep during conversation. He exhibits horizontal and vertical nystagmus and bilateral gaze palsies. Examination of the periphery reveals a symmetrical polyneuropathy. This diagnostic picture is most consistent with which of the following?

(A) Korsakoff's psychosis
(B) Marchiafava-Bignami disease
(C) Wernicke's disease
(D) Wernicke-Korsakoff syndrome
(E) Alcoholic hypoglycemia

458. A 10-year-old mentally retarded boy has developed a grand mal seizure disorder. On examination, a peculiar nodular appearance is noted over his cheeks and nose. His skull x-ray shows scattered intracerebral calcifications. His pneumoencephalogram demonstrates nodules on the surface of the lateral ventricles. The most likely diagnosis is

(A) Pick's disease
(B) cerebral palsy
(C) spastic pseudosclerosis
(D) ependymoma
(E) tuberous sclerosis

459. A diagnosis of acute idiopathic polyneuritis (Guillain-Barré syndrome) is most consistent with which of the following sets of cerebrospinal fluid values in a patient who has had a lumbar puncture after five days of illness?

	Glucose mg/100 ml	Protein mg/100 ml	Cells /mm^3
(A)	10	20	2
(B)	20	100	100
(C)	80	20	10
(D)	80	60	0
(E)	80	500	0

460. The drug most effective in the treatment of tic douloureux (trigeminal neuralgia) is

(A) phenytoin (Dilantin)
(B) carbamazepine
(C) prednisone
(D) pentazocine
(E) thiamine hydrochloride

461. A 55-year-old diabetic woman suddenly develops weakness of the left side of her face as well as of her right arm and leg. She also has diplopia on left lateral gaze. The lesion affecting this patient is probably located in the

(A) right cerebral hemisphere
(B) left cerebral hemisphere
(C) right side of the brain stem
(D) left side of the brain stem
(E) right medial longitudinal fasciculus

462. A 67-year-old woman is sitting watching television when suddenly she complains of a severe headache. She then vomits and over the next few minutes slips into a coma. The patient has probably suffered which of the following cerebrovascular accidents?

(A) Ruptured mycotic aneurysm
(B) Cerebral embolism
(C) Cerebral thrombosis
(D) Cerebral hemorrhage
(E) Subdural hematoma

463. It is frequently difficult to distinguish between early bacterial meningitis and early viral meningitis. In ascertaining the diagnosis of bacterial meningitis, which of the following cerebrospinal fluid indices would be of greatest help?

(A) Leukocyte count
(B) Ratio of polymorphonuclear to mononuclear leukocytes
(C) Glucose level
(D) Protein level
(E) Pressure

DIRECTIONS: Each question below contains four suggested answers of which **one** or **more** is correct. Choose the answer:

A	if	**1, 2, and 3**	are correct
B	if	**1 and 3**	are correct
C	if	**2 and 4**	are correct
D	if	**4**	is correct
E	if	**1, 2, 3, and 4**	are correct

464. Peripheral neuropathy has been associated with which of the following drugs?

(1) Nitrofurantoin
(2) Vincristine
(3) Isoniazid
(4) Stilbamidine

465. Correct statements concerning multiple sclerosis include which of the following?

(1) Optic neuritis is a common presenting manifestation
(2) Seizures occur in approximately 40 percent of patients over the course of the disease
(3) The disease is very rare between latitudes 35° north and south
(4) Peripheral nerve involvement with absent reflexes may occur

466. Bitemporal hemianopia is commonly associated with which of the following conditions?

(1) Craniopharyngioma
(2) Multiple sclerosis
(3) Aneurysm of the circle of Willis
(4) Methyl alcohol poisoning

467. In typical (idiopathic) Bell's palsy, patients often manifest which of the following signs?

(1) Paralysis of one side of the mouth
(2) Decreased sensitivity to noise in the ipsilateral ear
(3) Loss of taste sensitivity on one side of the tongue anteriorly
(4) Inability to open fully the ipsilateral eye

468. A 14-year-old boy has a port-wine hemangioma on the right side of his forehead and a left hemiparesis. He is also likely to have which of the following associated manifestations?

(1) Calcifications on skull x-ray
(2) Seizures
(3) Mental retardation
(4) Right arm and leg hemiatrophy

469. Cerebral thrombosis may be caused by which of the following diseases?

(1) Atherosclerosis
(2) Systemic lupus erythematosus
(3) Polycythemia
(4) Syphilis

470. In older individuals, amyotrophic lateral sclerosis and cervical spondylosis may mimic each other. Laboratory tests that help to distinguish these disorders include

(1) nerve conduction velocity
(2) electromyography
(3) cerebrospinal fluid protein electrophoresis
(4) myelography

DIRECTIONS: The groups of questions below consist of lettered choices followed by several numbered items. For each numbered item select the **one** lettered choice with which it is **most** closely associated. Each lettered choice may be used once, more than once, or not at all.

Questions 471-474

For each of the following clinical findings, select the disease with which it is most closely associated.

(A) Duchenne dystrophy
(B) Limb-girdle dystrophy
(C) Peroneal muscular atrophy
(D) Myotonic dystrophy (atrophy)
(E) Polymyositis

471. Absent Achilles reflexes

472. Enlargement of the gastrocnemius muscles

473. Elevated erythrocyte sedimentation rate

474. Atrophy of temporalis and facial muscles

Questions 475-478

For each of the following complexes of neurologic findings, select the disorder with which it is most closely related.

(A) Poliomyelitis
(B) Amyotrophic lateral sclerosis
(C) Pernicious anemia
(D) Multiple sclerosis
(E) Cervical spondylosis

475. Asymmetric motor, sensory, and bladder symptoms, each developing at a different time

476. Asymmetric muscle atrophy and loss of deep tendon reflexes in one leg

477. Spasticity and loss of vibration in the legs, with radicular pain and muscle atrophy in one arm

478. Fairly symmetric muscle atrophy and hyperreflexia of the arms and legs, with sensory function intact

Neurology
Answers

450. The answer is C. *(Isselbacher, ed 9. pp 354-355. Merritt, ed 6. pp 628-629.)* The most likely diagnosis for the patient presented in the question is temporal arteritis, an illness that usually affects elderly individuals. Systemic symptoms may include fever, anorexia, and sweats. Immediate steroid therapy is indicated if there are no serious contraindications. Analgesia, anticoagulation, and antiplatelet therapy are not sufficient because these modes of therapy do not attack the primary problem, which is an inflammatory arteritis. Consequently, such measures cannot prevent the most serious complication, which is arterial occlusion.

451. The answer is E. *(Isselbacher, ed 9. pp 46, 400, 2002, 2018.)* Vitamin B_{12} deficiency, apart from producing pernicious anemia, affects the nervous system, characteristically producing a subacute combined degeneration of the spinal cord, involving posterior column and pyramidal tract lesions. Peripheral neuropathy occurs in addition. Multiple disc lesions, particularly those that occur at the L5-S1 region in combination with defects above this level, may cause a myelopathy. Progressive degeneration of unknown etiology of motor neurons may occur in the cerebral cortex, brain stem, and spinal cord, or any combination thereof. Such degeneration usually is grouped under the heading of motor neuron disease or motor system disease. Depending on the areas of the nervous system predominantly involved, subdivisions can be recognized. The most commonly occurring form of motor system disease, associated with muscular atrophy and hyperreflexia, is amyotrophic lateral sclerosis. A progressive muscular atrophy and progressive bulbar palsy, together with primary lateral sclerosis, can also present a distinctive syndrome. Both motor system disease and syringomyelia may give rise to upper motor neuron lesions and to a lower motor neuron lesion at the L5-S1 nerve root, thus producing the upper motor neuron sign of extensor plantar reflexes and the lower motor neuron sign of absent ankle reflexes. A tumor of the cauda equina, which occurs below the end of the upper motor neurons, thus cannot produce extensor plantar reflexes.

452. The answer is B. *(Isselbacher, ed 9. pp 1749-1750. Tower, vol 2. p 198.)* Rapid correction of severe hyperglycemia leads to a prompt drop in plasma osmolality resulting from the drastic blood glucose reduction. These changes produce an osmotic shift of water into the central nervous system, which also will have become hyperosmolar during the development of the underlying hyperglycemia. This movement of water into the central nervous system causes cerebral edema and mental deterioration.

453. The answer is D. *(Isselbacher, ed 9. pp 203, 2049. Merritt, ed 6. pp 356-363.)* The fifth lumbar root leaves the spine between the fifth lumbar and first sacral vertebrae. Thus, herniation of the disc between L5 and S1 spares that root, but compresses the first sacral root, which leaves the spine through the first sacral foramen. Such herniation produces numbness of the ipsilateral calf and foot, as well as loss of the ankle jerk. The L5-S1 disc is the most common to herniate.

454. The answer is D. *(Isselbacher, ed 9. p 2007. Merritt, ed 6. pp 248-253.)* Acoustic neuromas account for 5 to 10 percent of intracranial tumors. They are slow growing and rarely cause symptoms before the third decade of life. Acoustic neuromas classically produce hearing loss and impaired vestibular function (decreased caloric responsiveness), as well as an elevated cerebrospinal fluid protein level (above 45 mg/100 ml). Nystagmus is present in almost all cases. Meniere's disease produces hearing and vestibular dysfunction but not elevated cerebrospinal fluid protein. Labyrinthitis and vestibular neuronitis do not impair hearing.

455. The answer is E. *(Isselbacher, ed 9. pp 117, 119. Tower, vol 2. pp 78-80.)* Patients in coma following drug intoxication have a fairly good chance of full recovery, provided they are still breathing by the time help is available. Extreme hypothermia, especially in combination with a mild intoxication, may also produce a comatose condition that is reversible. No other causes for coma have been associated with a reasonable chance of full recovery.

456. The answer is E. *(Isselbacher, ed 9. p 113. Merritt, ed 6. pp 710-715.)* Position and vibration sense from the feet are transmitted in the posterior columns of the spinal cord. Hyperreflexia of the legs and bilateral Babinski signs are an indication of pyramidal tract disease involving the lateral columns of the spinal cord. Thus, a person who has impairment of position and vibration sense, as well as pyramidal tract signs, has a lesion that involves the lateral and posterior columns of the spinal cord.

457. The answer is C. *(Isselbacher, ed 9. pp 1985-1987.)* Wernicke's disease, as exemplified in the patient presented in the question, is characterized by ocular disturbances consisting of (1) weakness or paralysis of external recti, (2) nystagmus, and (3) various paralyses of conjugate gaze. Ataxia and a global confusion state also are characteristic. In more than 80 percent of affected patients, polyneuropathy occurs. Korsakoff's psychosis, known also as the amnesia-confabulatory syndrome, is not a separate disease but a variably present psychic component of Wernicke's disease involving impairment of retentive memory and learning ability. When both neurological and psychic elements of the disease are present, it is known as the Wernicke-Korsakoff syndrome. Marchiafava-Bignami disease, which is limited to Italian men who are heavy wine drinkers, is associated with bilateral demyelinization of the corpus callosum; clinically, this disease is characterized by (1) emotional disorders, (2) loss of mental faculties, (3) convulsions, and (4) a variety of motor disabilities.

458. The answer is E. *(Isselbacher, ed 9. p 207. Merritt, ed 6. pp 453-460.)* Tuberous sclerosis, a familial disease characterized by congenital tumors that develop during childhood, causes progressive mental deterioration and convulsions. In addition to a variety of central nervous system lesions, the disease classically is associated with facial nevi and also may cause tumors of the eye (phakomas) and other organs (especially the kidneys and the heart). There is no specific treatment for the condition; the average life span of affected patients is less than 15 years.

459. The answer is D. *(Isselbacher, ed 9. p 2029.)* The classical finding in Guillain-Barré syndrome is acellular cerebrospinal fluid (CSF) under normal pressure. CSF glucose levels are normal. Most affected patients exhibit an elevation of CSF protein after the first few days of the disease. In a small fraction of these patients, a pleocytosis (predominantly lymphocytes and mononuclear cells) of up to 50 cells/mm^3, occasionally as high as 200 cells/mm^3, is found. However, the dissociation of protein and cells is characteristic of this syndrome.

460. The answer is B. *(Isselbacher, ed 9. p 2023. Merritt, ed 6. pp 380-383.)* The etiology of tic douloureux (trigeminal neuralgia) is unknown. The severe, lancinating pain characterizing this disorder may occur in other conditions such as temperomandibular joint disease. Carbamazepine is now the drug of choice for treatment of this condition, and is effective in most patients. Phenytoin (Dilantin) is also helpful. Less specific types of treatment, such as corticosteroids, have not been particularly helpful in this condition. Attempts at surgical relief for this syndrome, such as root decompression and partial nerve section, have achieved mixed results.

461. The answer is D. *(Isselbacher, ed 9. pp 89, 1921. Merritt, ed 6. pp 193-195.)* The diabetic patient described in the question has weakness of one side of a cranial structure, in this instance the face, and weakness of the opposite side of the body, in this instance the right arm and leg. This "crossed hemiplegia" is characteristic of brain stem lesions. The cranial nerve nuclei, of course, are ipsilateral to the structures that their nerves innervate; in this patient, it is the left sixth and seventh cranial nerves that are affected. However, because her lesion is **above** the level of decussation of the pyramidal tract, the arm and leg **contralateral** to the lesion site are affected.

462. The answer is D. *(Isselbacher, ed 9. pp 1932-1937. Merritt, ed 6. pp 158-161.)* In older individuals, rupture of an arteriosclerotic artery with cerebral hemorrhage is the most common cause of a sudden headache that is followed by vomiting and terminates in coma. This progression to coma is fairly frequent in cerebral hemorrhage and less common in cerebral embolism or thrombosis. Subdural hematoma also may produce headache and coma, but rarely so precipitately as in the patient described in the question.

463. The answer is C. *(Isselbacher, ed 9. pp 1960-1963. Merritt, ed 6. pp 1-9.)* In both early bacterial and viral meningitis, the cerebrospinal fluid may have an elevated white blood cell count with predominantly polymorphonuclear forms; the pressure and protein levels also may be mildly elevated. However, only in bacterial meningitis is the glucose content significantly depressed, i.e., usually below 20 mg/100 ml.

464. The answer is E (all). *(Isselbacher, ed 9. p 2028.)* Peripheral neuropathy has been associated with all the drugs listed in the question. Paresthesia of the toes and feet followed by similar sensory changes in the fingers are the early symptoms of nitrofurantoin neurotoxicity. If the drug is not discontinued after the onset of these symptoms, severe polyneuropathy may result. Generally, the neurotoxicity appears only after high dosage administration over several weeks or months. Patients with chronic renal failure are notably prone to this side effect. Vincristine causes a predominantly sensory polyneuropathy, as do stilbamidine and isoniazid. Isoniazid neurotoxicity is thought to be due to pyridoxine deficiency, and pyridoxine is administered with isoniazid for this reason.

465. The answer is B (1, 3). *(Isselbacher, ed 9. pp 1973-1974.)* Multiple sclerosis is a chronic neurological disease characterized by recurrent episodes—over a period of 20-30 years—of optic neuritis and symptoms due to brain stem and spinal cord involvement. Seizures, however, occur in only about five percent of affected patients. In multiple sclerosis, the central nervous system is always involved and the peripheral nerves are not. The disease is rarely found between latitudes 35° north and south. Persons who migrate from high risk to low risk areas retain their susceptibility to multiple sclerosis.

466. The answer is B (1, 3). *(Isselbacher, ed 9. p 2022.)* Pituitary adenoma, craniopharyngioma, and aneurysm of the circle of Willis all occur in close proximity to the optic chiasm, with involvement of the decussating nasal fibers from each retina. The field defect (bitemporal hemianopia) is often asymmetrical and may involve upper quadrants. Methyl alcohol, in contrast, causes bilateral scotomata, with central visual field defects. Multiple sclerosis, although a frequent cause of retrobulbar neuritis, does not cause this field defect with any frequency.

467. The answer is B (1, 3). *(Isselbacher, ed 9. pp 2023-2024. Merritt, ed 6. pp 384-385.)* Paralysis of the seventh facial nerve without a known cause is referred to as Bell's palsy and is presumed to be due to an inflammatory reaction of the nerve within the fallopian canal. Bell's palsy causes weakness of one side of the face and frequently a loss of taste in the ipsilateral anterior two-thirds of the tongue. The ipsilateral ear is often hypersensitive to noise—not hyposensitive. The ipsilateral eye may remain open due to muscular weakness of the orbicularis oculi, and an affected patient might thus be unable to fully close that eye.

468. The answer is A (1, 2, 3). *(Isselbacher, ed 9. p 2008. Merritt, ed 6. p 236.)* A port-wine hemangioma on one side of the forehead in conjunction with a contralateral hemiparesis is virtually pathognomic of Sturge-Weber disease. Calcifications on skull x-ray, as well as seizures and mental retardation, are commonly associated with this disorder. Because in the patient discussed in the question the hemiparesis is on the left, he might have a left arm and leg hemiatrophy, but not a right one. Anticonvulsants may help to control seizures; intractable epilepsy, however, may require hemispherectomy.

469. The answer is E (all). *(Isselbacher, ed 9. pp 1913-1929. Merritt, ed 6. pp 345-346.)* Cerebral thrombosis has myriad causes, including atherosclerosis, systemic lupus erythematosus, polycythemia, and syphilis. All these conditions involve either narrowing of arteries or sludging of blood cells. The obstruction produced by a thrombus may lead to cerebral infarction resulting in hemiplegia and loss of consciousness, or merely to exceedingly mild neurologic symptoms, depending upon the extent and location of the infarct.

470. The answer is C (2, 4). *(Isselbacher, ed 9. pp 2002, 2059. Merritt, ed 6. pp 549-559.)* The tests commonly employed to help distinguish amyotrophic lateral sclerosis (ALS) from cervical spondylosis are electromyography and myelography. Electromyography may disclose involvement of anterior horn cells outside the cervical region, thus favoring the diagnosis of ALS. Myelography may demonstrate a compressive lesion of the cervical spinal cord, thus pointing to cervical spondylosis.

471-474. The answers are: 471-C, 472-A, 473-E, 474-D. *(Isselbacher, ed 9. pp 2035, 2054, 2060-2061. Merritt, ed 6. pp 569, 580, 590, 636.)* Distal deep tendon reflexes disappear early in the course of a polyneuropathy that involves large myelinated fibers. An example of such loss of tendon reflexes is peroneal muscular atrophy. Muscle diseases, per se, generally do not compromise deep tendon reflexes until affected patients experience profound weakness.

"Pseudohypertrophy" of the calves is primarily associated with Duchenne dystrophy. This condition is the result of fat deposition in the muscle. While it may occur in other forms of dystrophy, gastrocnemius "hypertrophy" is rarely so striking as in Duchenne dystrophy.

A high erythrocyte sedimentation rate (ESR) is a classic sign of inflammation. Thus, the muscle disease that is characterized by inflammation would be expected to have an elevated ESR. For this reason, polymyositis and a high ESR are commonly linked, since polymyositis is an inflammatory myopathy.

Facial and temporalis muscle atrophy is characteristic of myotonic dystrophy (atrophy). Other muscles such as those in the forearm and hand also are wasted in this disease. Other myopathies, such as facioscapulohumeral muscular dystrophy, also can result in wasting of these same muscles.

475-478. The answers are: 475-D, 476-A, 477-E, 478-B. *(Isselbacher, ed 9. pp 812-813, 1974-1975, 2002, 2016-2017. McAlpine, ed 2. p 135. Merritt, ed 6. pp 58-63, 549, 734, 737.)* Multiple sclerosis produces a combination of motor, sensory, bladder, and cranial nerve symptoms. They usually occur asymmetrically, affecting different parts of the central nervous system with each attack. The less common, slowly progressive form of the disease also affects different structures at different times.

Poliomyelitis produces asymmetric muscle atrophy and loss of deep tendon reflexes, sometimes confined to one limb. The feature of polio that would separate it from a neuropathy or radiculopathy is the complete absence of sensory loss. While amyotrophic lateral sclerosis also may produce asymmetric muscle atrophy and loss of some deep tendon reflexes, hyperreflexia commonly exists in this disease, and it usually involves more than one limb.

Cervical spondylosis is a condition in which both cervical root compression and spinal cord compression may occur. The spinal cord compression will produce long tract signs including spasticity and loss of vibration sense in the legs. The root compression in the neck will produce radicular pain and muscle atrophy in the arms.

Amyotrophic lateral sclerosis, a degeneration of anterior horn cells, results in muscle atrophy that may be fairly symmetric. There also is degeneration of cortical neurons in the motor areas, along with their descending tracts, a process that produces hyperreflexia. The sensory examination should be essentially normal in patients who have amyotrophic lateral sclerosis.

Dermatology

DIRECTIONS: Each question below contains five suggested answers. Choose the **one best** response to each question.

479. Generalized exfoliative dermatitis is caused by which of the following disorders?

(A) Erythema multiforme
(B) Pemphigus vulgaris
(C) Mycosis fungoides
(D) Angiokeratoma corporis diffusum
(E) Atrophoderma of Pasini and Pierini

480. Whitish discoloration on the vaginal mucosa and vulva may be caused by all the following disorders EXCEPT

(A) extramammary Paget's disease
(B) leukoplakia
(C) lichen sclerosus et atrophicus
(D) vitiligo
(E) Behçet's syndrome

481. The squamous cell carcinoma that is LEAST aggressive and usually can be removed by simple excision arises from

(A) normal skin
(B) a mucocutaneous junction
(C) a burn scar
(D) a radiation burn
(E) an actinic keratosis

482. A 28-year-old woman who is three months postpartum notes a distressing loss of scalp hair. A meticulous physical examination is unremarkable; the scalp and hair appear normal, and there are no bald spots. The patient takes no medications and says that she feels well. The most likely cause of hair loss is

(A) postpartum hypothyroidism
(B) postpartum telogen effluvium
(C) hypervitaminosis due to vitamin supplementation during pregnancy
(D) trichotillomania
(E) alopecia areata

483. Erythema multiforme is caused by all the following EXCEPT

(A) sulfonamide drugs
(B) *Sarcoptes scabiei*
(C) *Mycoplasma pneumoniae*
(D) herpes simplex
(E) histoplasmosis

484. Erythema multiforme may exhibit all the following clinical findings EXCEPT

(A) hair loss
(B) petechiae
(C) urticaria
(D) blisters
(E) mouth erosions

485. A young woman has recurrent episodes, lasting one to two weeks, of very painful ulcers scattered over the labial and buccal mucosa and occasionally on the pharynx. No blisters appear. Her lesions have no apparent association with stress, fever, or menses. The oval ulcers are 1 to 2 mm in size with a gray base and red border. The most likely diagnosis is

(A) herpes simplex
(B) herpes zoster
(C) aphthous stomatitis
(D) contact dermatitis
(E) desquamative gingivitis

486. A febrile patient receiving penicillin for streptococcal pharyngitis develops showers of 3 to 4 mm purpuric spots on the legs. Most of the lesions are raised and palpable. The most likely diagnosis is

(A) erythema nodosum
(B) erythema induratum
(C) Weber-Christian syndrome
(D) allergic angiitis
(E) thrombocytopenia

487. Diabetes mellitus is associated with all the following cutaneous signs EXCEPT

(A) granuloma annulare
(B) necrobiosis lipoidica
(C) lipoatrophy
(D) brown atrophic macules on the pretibial surface
(E) lichen simplex chronicus

488. A three-year-old girl has six or seven oval white spots on her trunk. She has pink papules at the nasolabial folds and on her cheeks. Her parents should be advised that their daughter

(A) has infantile acne and should be treated with tetracycline and vitamin A acid
(B) should have the papules removed by dermabrasion because they will enlarge and become cosmetically disfiguring
(C) needs careful observation by a gastroenterologist because of the high probability of malignancy of the colon
(D) needs careful observation by a neurologist because of the high probability of seizures or mental retardation
(E) needs careful observation by a cardiologist because of the high probability of cardiovascular disease

489. A 78-year-old derelict man is hospitalized for an acute myocardial infarction. On physical examination, he is found to have coiled hairs and a petechial rash distributed around the hair follicles. These abnormalities are most obvious in the groin and thighs. The patient's gums are bloody. The most probable cause of this man's skin lesions is

(A) leukemia cutis
(B) thrombocytopenia
(C) kwashiorkor
(D) vitamin C deficiency
(E) niacin deficiency

490. Sarcoidosis is associated with all the following cutaneous signs EXCEPT

(A) hair loss
(B) red plaques
(C) "carpet tack" scales
(D) erythema nodosum
(E) waxy, pigmented papules

491. Generalized pruritus without diagnostic skin lesions occurs in all the following conditions EXCEPT

(A) hyperthyroidism
(B) polycythemia vera
(C) carcinoid syndrome
(D) secondary syphilis
(E) pregnancy

492. Psoriasis is characterized by all the following statements EXCEPT that

(A) it affects more than 2 percent of the population
(B) lesions rarely occur on the scalp
(C) it consists of isolated scaling papules or plaques
(D) the borders of the plaques are distinct
(E) the plaques are pink to deep red

493. Psoralens, of which methoxsalen is an example, are being increasingly used in the treatment of skin disease. They are effective in all the following diseases EXCEPT

(A) psoriasis
(B) vitiligo
(C) eczema
(D) mycosis fungoides
(E) porphyria cutanea tarda

494. Herpes zoster (shingles) is characterized by all the following statements EXCEPT that it

(A) is caused by varicella virus
(B) typically produces a few scattered vesicles
(C) has a high rate of recurrence
(D) is not contagious for individuals who have had chickenpox
(E) has a significant association with malignant lymphoma

495. For most patients who have acute acne, which of the following drugs is the agent of choice?

(A) Retinoic acid
(B) Oral clindamycin
(C) Topical clindamycin
(D) Benzoyl peroxide
(E) Aluminum chloride hexahydrate

496. Exfoliative dermatitis is characterized by all the following statements EXCEPT that it

(A) can occur as a result of a pre-existing dermatitis
(B) occurs in association with lymphoma
(C) may involve all of the skin surface
(D) is a scaling, erythematous lesion
(E) is associated with a 10 percent mortality

497. An obviously ill two-year-old child is brought to a pediatrician. The parents are frantic. The child has had a runny, crusted nose for one week and a low grade fever. Twenty-four hours previously his skin became red and tender; it is now peeling off in sheets. Examination confirms that the child's skin is shedding, very red, and tender. He also has purulent conjunctivitis. He has received no medications. The pediatrician concludes that the child

(A) should be admitted to the hospital burn unit and receive intravenous prednisone, 40 mg daily in divided doses
(B) should be placed in protective isolation and started on prophylactic antibiotics
(C) has late onset epidermolysis bullosa dystrophica, which will cause severe scarring
(D) has a toxic reaction to the products of *Staphylococcus aureus,* undoubtedly the cause of his purulent conjunctivitis
(E) has Stevens-Johnson syndrome due to a virus infection, and should receive steroids to avert ocular scarring and blindness

498. A patient receiving thiazide diuretics or sulfonamides who is subject to photosensitive drug reactions may use all the following sunscreens EXCEPT

(A) benzophenones
(B) zinc oxide
(C) titanium oxide
(D) kaolin
(E) para-aminobenzoic acid (PABA)

499. A 39-year-old woman has had nonhealing painful erosions in her mouth for the past year. She now observes rapidly spreading blisters on her chest and erosions of her scalp; the lesions are flaccid and red at the base. A biopsy report notes acantholysis of the prickle cells and deposition of IgG and complement in the intercellular spaces of the epidermis. Which of the following statements best summarizes both this woman's disorder and the appropriate treatment?

(A) She has a blistering disorder curable only by the most potent topical steroids, e.g., 0.5% triamcinolone (Aristocort) applied every two to three hours
(B) She has an autoimmune disorder and should be treated with 6-mercaptopurine or methotrexate
(C) She has a disease that is fatal unless treated with prednisone 100 mg or more daily
(D) She has cutaneous lupus erythematosus and should receive oral hydroxychloroquine, 400 mg a day
(E) She has bullous impetigo and needs oral penicillinase-resistant antibiotics for 7 to 10 days

DIRECTIONS: The question below contains four suggested answers of which **one** or **more** is correct. Choose the answer:

A	if	**1, 2, and 3**	are correct
B	if	**1 and 3**	are correct
C	if	**2 and 4**	are correct
D	if	**4**	is correct
E	if	**1, 2, 3, and 4**	are correct

500. A 39-year-old woman afflicted with vitiligo is likely to have a personal or family history of which of the following diseases?

(1) Hashimoto's thyroiditis
(2) Graves' disease
(3) Pernicious anemia
(4) Diabetes mellitus

Dermatology
Answers

479. The answer is C. *(Isselbacher, ed 9. p 1654.)* Mycosis fungoides, a lymphoma of the skin, can pass through several stages. The first is a diffuse erythroderma and exfoliative dermatitis. In the second phase, plaques develop, and in the third phase, tumors and nodules are found. Not everyone who has exfoliative dermatitis has mycosis fungoides. Exfoliative dermatitis has other causes such as psoriasis, drug reactions, seborrheic dermatitis, and pityriasis rubra pilaris. Erythema multiforme and pemphigus produce blisters. Angiokeratoma corporis diffusum (Fabry's disease) exhibits unusual capillaries in the skin, especially in the groin and eye, and may cause fatal renal disease. Atrophoderma of Pasini and Pierini is an atrophic disease virtually impossible to confuse with an erythroderma.

480. The answer is E. *(Braverman, p 8. Isselbacher, ed 9. pp 1886-1887.)* Whitish patches on the vulva or vaginal mucosa must suggest extramammary Paget's disease as well as leukoplakia, lichen sclerosus et atrophicus, and vitiligo. The whitish color is present in each disease for a completely different reason. Behçet's syndrome produces aphthous ulcers of the mouth and vagina, and often changes in the eye. Vitiligo is caused by a loss of pigment cells, leaving white skin and mucous membranes.

481. The answer is E. *(Isselbacher, ed 9. p 1653.)* The sun-induced squamous cell carcinoma, which has a very low potential for metastasis, is easily removed by simple excision or even by topical 5-fluorouracil. In contrast, the other four squamous cell carcinomas listed in the question metastasize quickly and require vigorous excision and follow-up.

482. The answer is B. *(Domonkos, ed 6. p 2840.)* In the patient presented in the question, the most probable cause of hair loss is normal postpartum telogen effluvium. In the first trimester of pregnancy, telogen hairs (resting hairs) constitute a normal 15 to 20 percent of all hair; later in pregnancy, the telogen hair count may drop to 10 percent. This means that many follicles that normally would have reached the end of their active (anagen) phase are still present at parturition. Telogen counts rise quickly in the postpartum period, sometimes reaching 30 to 40 percent of total hair. Telogen lasts approximately three months. At the end of this period, there is abnormally heavy shedding while a normal telogen-to-anagen hair ratio is reestablished. A patient who presents with hair loss should be carefully examined for circular bald spots that might indicate alopecia areata or trichotillomania. Trichotillomania, which is loss of hair from pulling, usually causes bald areas with severed hair roots at their bases. Hypothyroidism and hypervitaminoses can both cause alopecia, but there is no reason to suspect them in this patient.

483. The answer is B. *(Braverman, pp 256-261. Isselbacher, ed 9. p 919.)* Drugs are a common cause of erythema multiforme, as are infections, including all those listed in the question except that due to *Sarcoptes scabiei* (scabies). Erythema multiforme is thought to be a hypersensitivity syndrome, but the mechanism is unknown.

484. The answer is A. *(Braverman, pp 256-261. Isselbacher, ed 9. p 245.)* Hair loss does not occur with erythema multiforme. The early lesions associated with this disease include hives and superimposed petechiae or blisters, or both. Such combinations of dermatoses form target lesions that are the classic sign of erythema multiforme. The associated mouth lesions usually are blisters that have ruptured.

485. The answer is C. *(Isselbacher, ed 9. p 190.)* The patient presented in the question probably has aphthous ulcers, lesions that frequently are misdiagnosed as herpes simplex. Herpes tends to cause a group of shallow, round ulcers, frequently beginning as blisters and having a red or yellowish color at the base. These lesions can recur but usually not as often as aphthae. The cause of aphthae is unknown; repeated cultures for viruses, mycoplasmata, and other pathogens have been negative. Moreover, attempts to treat the lesions with antibiotics have been unsuccessful. Topical steroids seem to be equally ineffective. Topical anesthetics may provide symptomatic relief.

486. The answer is D. *(Isselbacher, ed 9. p 1323.)* The patient described in the question probably has allergic necrotizing angiitis, a lesion caused by trapping of circulating immune complexes under the basement membrane of the capillaries. The complexes attract neutrophils that promptly phagocytize them, releasing proteolytic enzymes that disrupt the capillaries and produce a palpable form of purpura. Erythema nodosum is usually not purpuric, but the lesions are larger than those exhibited by this patient. Erythema induratum has clinical characteristics similar to erythema nodosum. Weber-Christian syndrome is a panniculitis manifested as tender red plaques. Thrombocytopenia produces petechiae that are not raised. The lesions of allergic angiitis, however, are distinctly palpable, a singular quality that always should alert the physician to the probability of an allergic disorder. A biopsy from the skin can confirm the diagnosis.

487. The answer is E. *(Isselbacher, ed 9. pp 242, 1754.)* Lichen simplex is not associated with diabetes mellitus. Disseminated granuloma annulare, however, is frequently the first sign of the disease, and necrobiosis lipoidica diabeticorum and lipoatrophy are virtually pathognomonic signs. Atrophic brown macules, termed diabetic dermopathy, also are classic manifestations of diabetes.

488. The answer is D. *(Isselbacher, ed 9. p 2007.)* The girl described in the question has tuberous sclerosis. Ash-leaf spots (hypopigmented macules), especially occurring early in life, along with the pink papules (adenoma sebaceum) are dermatologically diagnostic of the disease. Calcification of the brain, periungual fibromas, and phakomas are other signs of tuberous sclerosis. Its worst effects are severe mental retardation and seizures. Occasionally, tumors arise in the brain (especially gliomas) and in the kidney, liver, and thyroid.

489. The answer is D. *(Isselbacher, ed 9. pp 429-430.)* The skin findings in the patient presented in the question are classic for scurvy. In the untreated disease, the hair follicles themselves become enlarged and red and, ultimately, hemorrhagic from the proliferation of surrounding blood vessels. None of the other diseases listed in the question produce similar manifestations.

490. The answer is C. *(Braverman, pp 274-275. Isselbacher, ed 9. p 931.)* "Carpet tack" scales are found in lupus erythematosus. The other dermal manifestations listed in the question are classic for sarcoidosis, especially red plaques and brown waxy papules; scarring alopecia unfortunately is another sign of this disorder. Occasionally, a patient who has sarcoidosis also develops erythema nodosum as a secondary manifestation.

491. The answer is D. *(Isselbacher, ed 9. pp 247-248.)* A number of conditions are characterized by a generalized pruritus in the absence of recognizable skin lesions. Hyperthyroidism, carcinoid syndrome, and pruritus of pregnancy often are associated with cholestasis, which may be overt; affected patients may manifest jaundice or merely an elevation of serum alkaline phosphatase and bile acids. Although syphilis causes a plethora of skin lesions—notably macules or papules in secondary syphilis—pruritus in the absence of skin lesions is extremely rare in patients who have syphilis.

492. The answer is B. *(Isselbacher, ed 9. pp 239, 256.)* Psoriatic lesions occur quite frequently on the scalp as well as on the elbows, knees, and sacrum. The scalp lesions are sharply demarcated, as are those on the rest of the skin. These sharply demarcated margins differentiate psoriasis from seborrheic dermatitis, which also commonly affects the scalp. Since the scales may be anchored by hair, they may "heap up" so that localized accumulations are usually felt. In contrast, seborrheic dermatitis does not produce this degree of accumulation; instead, it produces a diffuse, scaly erythema. Hair loss does not usually occur in psoriasis unless the hair is removed from excessive scratching of the lesions.

493. The answer is E. *(Isselbacher, ed 9. pp 261-262.)* Psoralens, used in conjunction with ultraviolet radiation UV-A (320-400 nm), are frequently employed in treating psoriasis. Psoralens also have been widely used in treating vitiligo, eczema, and mycosis fungoides. In the presence of psoralen, irradiation with ultraviolet A results in the binding of psoralens to pyrimidine bases in DNA. This reaction leads to inhibition of DNA synthesis followed by cell death. Methoxsalen is given in a dose range of 0.6-0.9 mg/kg. Patients who are candidates for this regimen are exposed to a measured dose of ultraviolet radiation following ingestion of the medication. Repeated psoralen-ultraviolet A treatment has been observed to cause disappearance of psoriatic lesions. Possible side effects of this and other types of photochemotherapy include premature aging, cataracts, and skin cancer.

494. The answer is C. *(Isselbacher, ed 9. p 802.)* Most patients who have herpes zoster (shingles) are basically healthy and remain so. However, the disease occurs in 25 percent of individuals who have lymphoma, Hodgkin's disease in particular. An affliction chiefly of adulthood, shingles arises from endogenous varicella virus that has lain dormant since the time of its original manifestation as chickenpox. Thus shingles—unlike chickenpox, which is caused by the same virus—is acquired not exogenously but from within. Children who have not been exposed to varicella-herpes zoster virus, when exposed to shingles, can develop chickenpox. There is no documented evidence that shingles is directly transmittable. Unlike herpes simplex, herpes zoster rarely recurs.

495. The answer is D. *(Melski, N Engl J Med 302:503-505, 1980.)* A wide range of effective topical agents is now available for the treatment of acne. The single most useful group of topical agents are the benzoyl peroxide preparations. Benzoyl peroxide has an antimicrobial effect, reducing free fatty acids and *P. acnes* bacteria effectively. Although contact irritation may occur with this agent, it is less than with retinoic acid. In addition, benzoyl peroxide may possess both sebostatic and comedolytic properties.

496. The answer is E. *(Isselbacher, ed 9. p 241.)* The course of exfoliative dermatitis is determined by its etiology: in patients with generalized skin disease—psoriasis, for example—the disease resolves itself, whereas in systemic disease such as lymphoma, the prognosis is relatively poor. Exfoliative dermatitis may occur as a result of a drug reaction, as a manifestation of a generalized pre-existing dermatitis, or in association with systemic disease such as lymphoma and leukemia. Approximately 60 percent of affected patients recover in less than a year; of the remaining, 10 percent have a persistent lesion that does not respond to treatment, and 30 percent die.

497. The answer is D. *(Elias, Arch Dermatol 113:207, 1977. Isselbacher, ed 9. p 610.)* The child presented in the question has toxic epidermal necrolysis (TEN), a relatively benign disease produced by a toxin released from certain *Staphylococcus aureus* organisms, group 2, phage-type 78. The syndrome is rarely lethal. The child should be treated with supportive fluids and dicloxacillin, and his parents with reassurance. Steroids are contraindicated, and no special burn therapy is required. Within a few days, the patient will be well. *Staphylococcus*-induced TEN, probably related to Ritter's disease, is different from drug-induced TEN, which usually occurs in adults and carries a very grim prognosis.

498. The answer is E. *(Isselbacher, ed 9. p 262.)* Sunscreens protect the skin by absorbing and reflecting radiation. Most sunscreens are formulated to protect against UV-B in the 290-320 nm range. The greatest protection is provided by 5 percent para-aminobenzoic acid (PABA) lotions. Drug-induced photosensitization reactions can be minimized by prescribing sunscreens containing benzophenones. PABA or its derivatives should not be prescribed for persons who are photosensitive to certain drugs, including thiazide diuretics and sulfonamides. In these patients, there may be a cross-reaction with PABA, leading to eczematous dermatitis. Such individuals should use benzophenones or opaque sunscreens containing zinc oxide and titanium oxide. Sunscreens containing light-scattering agents such as kaolin may also be used.

499. The answer is C. *(Isselbacher, ed 9. pp 240-241.)* The patient discussed in the question has an advanced stage of pemphigus vulgaris, a disease that is fatal unless properly treated with prednisone. The drug should be given orally, 100 mg daily or more. When affected patients have improved, the dose can be lowered and methotrexate can be added to minimize the need for oral steroids. However, low-dose steroids or immunosuppressive agents early in the course of pemphigus are often unavailing. Approximately 30 percent of patients having this disease die from complications of treatment; of the survivors, many eventually dispense with medication entirely and lead normal lives.

500. The answer is E (all). *(Braverman, pp 354, 369, 382. Isselbacher, ed 9. pp 251-253.)* Patients suffering from vitiligo have a high incidence of other disorders, especially of an autoimmune variety like those listed in the question. Even affected patients who do not have these disorders may have circulating antibodies against, for instance, the thyroid or islet cells. The cause of vitiligo is unknown; it is believed related in some manner to the immune system, although Lerner has hypothesized a neurogenic basis for the disease. Vitiligo is a hypomelanotic disorder that, while generally asymptomatic, may cause itching and burning on exposure to sunlight, its hypopigmented patches favoring skin areas that normally are highly endowed with pigment.

Bibliography

Acton JD, et al: *Fundamentals of Medical Virology: For Students of Medicine and Related Sciences.* Philadelphia, Lea & Febiger, 1974.

Almy TP, Howell DA: Diverticular disease of the colon. *N Engl J Med* 302:324-331, 1980.

Anderson T, Waldman TA, Javadpou RN, et al: Testicular germ cell between germ and cell neoplasms: recent advances in diagnosis and therapy. *Ann Intern Med* 90:373-385, 1979.

Anderson WAD, Kissane JM: *Pathology,* 7th ed. St. Louis, CV Mosby, 1977.

Arnett E, Roberts W: Acute infective endocarditis: a clinicopathologic analysis of 137 necropsy patients. *Curr Probl Cardiol* 1:11-18, 1976.

Bach JF (ed): *Immunology.* New York, John Wiley, 1977.

Barbour GL, Juniper K Jr: A clinical comparison of amebic and pyogenic abscess of the liver in sixty-six patients. *Am J Med* 53:323-334, 1972.

Bates DV, Macklem PT, Christie RV: *Respiratory Function in Disease,* 2nd ed. Philadelphia, WB Saunders, 1971.

Beeson PB, McDermott W, Wyngaarden JB: *Cecil Textbook of Medicine,* 15th ed. Philadelphia, WB Saunders, 1979.

Bellet S: *Essentials of Cardiac Arrhythmias: Diagnosis and Management.* Philadelphia, WB Saunders, 1972.

Benacerraf B: *Immunogenetics and Immunodeficiency.* Baltimore, University Park Press, 1975.

Benenson AS (ed): *Control of Communicable Disease in Man,* 12th ed. Washington, American Public Health Association, 1975.

Berman M, Alter HF, Ishak KG, et al: The chronic sequelae of non-A, non-B hepatitis. *Ann Intern Med* 91:1-6, 1979.

Blandy J: *Urology.* Philadelphia, JB Lippincott, 1976.

Blum RH, Carter SK, Agre K: A clinical review of bleomycin—a new anti-neoplastic agent. *Cancer* 31:903-914, 1973.

Bobrowitz ID: Ethambutol-INH vs. streptomycin-ethambutol-INH in original treatment of tuberculosis. *Am Rev Respir Dis* 109:548-553, 1974.

Bondy PK, Rosenberg LE: *Diseases of Metabolism,* 8th ed. Philadelphia, WB Saunders, 1979.

Bradley EL III, Clements JL, Gonzalez AC: The natural history of pancreatic pseudocysts: a unified concept of management. *Am J Surg* 137:135-141, 1979.

Braverman IM: *Skin Signs of Systemic Disease.* Philadelphia, WB Saunders, 1970.

Burrow GN, Ferris TF (eds): *Medical Complications During Pregnancy.* Philadelphia, WB Saunders, 1975.

Carpenter CC, Solomon N, Silverberg SC, et al: Schmidt's syndrome (thyroid and adrenal insufficiency): a review of the literature and a report of fifteen new cases including ten instances of coexistent diabetes mellitus. *Medicine* 43:153-180, 1964.

Chung EK: *Principles of Cardiac Arrhythmias,* 2nd ed. Baltimore, Williams & Wilkins, 1977.

Committee of the American Rheumatism Association Section of The Arthritis Foundation: Primer on the rheumatic diseases. *JAMA* 224(suppl):73-129, 1973.

Conn HW: Spontaneous peritonitis. *Gastroenterology* 70:455-457, 1976.

Conn HW, Fessel M: Spontaneous bacterial peritonitis in cirrhosis. *Medicine* 50:161-197, 1971.

Constant J: *Learning Electrocardiography: A Complete Course,* 2nd ed. Boston, Little, Brown, 1980.

Dienstag JL, Szmuness W, Stevens CE, et al: Hepatitis A virus infection: new insights from seroepidemiologic studies. *J Infect Dis* 137:328-340, 1978.

Domonkos AN: *Andrews' Diseases of the Skin,* 6th ed. Philadelphia, WB Saunders, 1971.

Downs JB, Klein EF Jr, Desautels D, et al: Intermittent mandatory ventilation: a new approach to weaning patients from mechanical ventilators. *Chest* 64: 331-335, 1973.

Dwyer JM: Identifying and enumerating human T and B lymphocytes. *Prog Allergy* 21:182-216, 1976.

Eisen HN: *Immunology.* Hagerstown, Harper & Row, 1974.

Elias PM, Fritsch P, Epstein EH: Staphylococcal scalded skin syndrome. Clinical features, pathogenesis, and recent microbiological and biochemical developments. *Arch Dermatol* 113:207-219, 1977.

Ellenberg M, Rifkin H: *Diabetes Mellitus: Theory and Practice.* New York, McGraw-Hill, 1970.

Finegold SM, Sutter VL: Susceptibility of gram negative anaerobic bacilli to gentamicin and other aminoglycosides. *J Infect Dis* 124 (suppl):56-58, 1971.

Forrester JS, Diamond G, Chatterjee K, et al: Medical therapy of acute myocardial infarction by application of hemodynamic subsets. *N Engl J Med* 295:1356-1360, 1976.

Freinkel N, Singer DL, Arky RA, et al: Alcohol hypoglycemia. I. Carbohydrate metabolism of patients with clinical alcohol hypoglycemia and the experimental reproduction of the syndrome with pure alcohol. *J Clin Invest* 42: 1112-1133, 1963.

Fudenberg HH, et al: *Basic and Clinical Immunology,* 2nd ed. Los Altos, Lange, 1978.

Gell PG, Coombs RR, Lachman PJ (eds): *Clinical Aspects of Immunology,* 3rd ed. Philadelphia, JB Lippincott, 1975.

Gordon EE, Kabadi UM: The hyperglycemic hyperosmolar syndrome. *Am J Med Sci* 271:252-268, 1976.

Hamilton CR, Maloof F: Unusual types of hyperthyroidism. *Medicine* 52:195-215, 1973.

Hammon W, Ho M: Viral encephalitis. *DM* February:31-35, 1973.

Hansten PD: *Drug Interactions,* 4th ed. Philadelphia, Lea & Febiger, 1979.

Harrison JH, et al, (eds): *Campbell's Urology,* 4th ed. Philadelphia, WB Saunders, 1978.

Heptinstall RH: *Pathology of the Kidney,* 2nd ed. Boston, Little, Brown, 1974.

Holland JF, Frei E, III: *Cancer Medicine.* Philadelphia, Lea & Febiger, 1973.

Hunt K: Diagnosis of hymenoptera hypersensitivity by skin testing with hymenoptera venoms. *J Allergy Clin Immunol* 59:2-8, 1977.

Hunter GW, Swartzwelder JC, Clyde DF (eds): *Tropical Medicine,* 5th ed. Philadelphia, WB Saunders, 1976.

Hurst JW, et al, (eds): *The Heart,* 4th ed. New York, McGraw-Hill, 1978.

Isbister JP: Plasmapheresis: a selective form of blood letting. *Med J Aust* 2: 167-170, 1979.

Isselbacher KJ, et al, (eds): *Harrison's Principles of Internal Medicine,* 9th ed. New York, McGraw-Hill, 1980.

Karandanis D: Factors associated with mortality in brain abscess. *Arch Intern Med* 135:1145-1149, 1975.

Kaye D: *Infective Endocarditis.* Baltimore, University Park Press, 1976.

Klein RG, Hunder GG, Stanson AW, et al: Large artery involvement in giant cell (temporal) arteritis. *Ann Intern Med* 83:806-812, 1975.

Klint CR, Knatterud GF, Meinert CL, et al: A study of the effects of hypoglycemic agents on vascular complications in patients with adult onset diabetes. *Diabetes* 19:747-830, 1970.

Knatterud CL, Klint CR, Osborne RK, et al: A study of the effects of hypoglycemic agents on vascular complications in patients with adult-onset diabetes. V. Evaluation of phenformin therapy. *Diabetes* 24:64-184, 1975.

Knight V: Influenza. *DM* August:27, 1976.

Kohler PF: Inherited complement deficiencies and systemic lupus erythematosus: an immunogenetic puzzle. *Ann Intern Med* 82:420-421, 1975.

Kohner M, Oakley NW: Diabetic retinopathy. *Metabolism* 24:1085-1098, 1976.

Kreisberg RA: Diabetic ketoacidosis: new concepts and trends in pathogenesis and treatment. *Ann Intern Med* 88:681-695, 1978.

Kucers A: *The Use of Antibiotics: A Comprehensive Review with Clinical Emphasis*, 3rd ed. Philadelphia, JB Lippincott, 1979.

Lerner AM, Jankauskas K: The classic bacterial pneumonias. *DM* February:22, 1975.

Levy RI: Hyperlipoproteinemia: concepts of diagnosis and management. *Curr Probl Cardiol* 1:23-24, 1976.

Lichstein E, Ribas-Meneclier C, Gupta P, et al: Incidence and description of accelerated ventricular rhythm complicating acute myocardial infarction. *Am J Med* 58:192-198, 1975.

MacKay IR: A survey of autoimmunity. *Postgrad Med* 35:7-17, 1969.

Mason DT: *Congestive Heart Failure.* New York, Yorke Medical, 1976.

Mathiason DA: Hypersensitivity to nonsteroidal drugs: indications and methods for oral challenges. *J Allergy Clin Immunol* 64:669-674, 1979.

McAlpine D, Lumsden CE, Acheson ED: *Multiple Sclerosis: A Reappraisal*, 2nd ed. New York, Longman, 1972.

McCarty DJ Jr (ed): *Arthritis and Allied Conditions: A Textbook of Rheumatology,* 9th ed. Philadelphia, Lea & Febiger, 1979.

Melski JW, Arndt KA: Current concepts: topical therapy for acne. *N Engl J Med* 302:503-505, 1980.

Merritt HH (ed): *Textbook of Neurology,* 6th ed. Philadelphia, Lea & Febiger, 1979.

Miller DJ: A case of a needle stick. *J Clin Gastroenterol* 1:251-258, 1979.

Miller M, Dalakos T, Moses AM, et al: Recognition of partial defects in antidiuretic hormone secretion. *Ann Intern Med* 73:721-729, 1970.

Moellering RC Jr, Swartz MN: Drug therapy: the newer cephalosporins. *N Engl J Med* 294:24-28, 1976.

Page MM, Alberti KG, Greenwood R, et al: Treatment of diabetic coma with continuous low-dose infusion of insulin. *Br Med J* 2:687-690, 1974.

Park BH, Good RA: *Principles of Modern Immunobiology: Basic and Clinical.* Philadelphia, Lea & Febiger, 1974.

Perloff JK: *The Clinical Recognition of Congenital Heart Disease,* 2nd ed. Philadelphia, WB Saunders, 1978.

Pollack EW, Michas CA, Wolfman EF Jr: Pancreatic pseudocyst: management in 54 patients. *Am J Surg* 135:199-201, 1978.

Powell LW, Bassett ML, Halliday JW: Hemochromatosis: 1980 update. *Gastroenterology* 78:374-381, 1980.

Priebe HJ, Skillman JJ, Bushnell LS, et al: Antacid vs. cimetidine in preventing acute gastrointestinal bleeding. A randomized trial in 75 critically ill patients. *N Engl J Med* 302:426-430, 1980.

Reduto LA, Gulotta SJ: Cardiology: prolapsed mitral valve syndrome. *Postgrad Med* 60:171-176, 1976.

Rotman M, Wagner GS, Wallace AG: Bradyarrhythmias in acute myocardial infarction. *Circulation* 45:703-722, 1972.

Samet P: *Cardiac Pacing,* 2nd ed. New York, Grune & Stratton, 1979.

Samter M: *Immunological Diseases,* 3rd ed. Boston, Little, Brown, 1978.

Savoie JC, Massin JP, Thomopoulos P, et al: Iodine induced thyrotoxicosis in apparently normal thyroid glands. *J Clin Endocrinol Metab* 41:685-691, 1975.

Schiff L: *Diseases of the Liver,* 4th ed. Philadelphia, JB Lippincott, 1975.

Selawry OS, Straus MJ: Lung cancer. *Semin Oncol* 1:163-287, 1974.

Sherlock S: *Diseases of the Liver and Biliary System,* 5th ed. Philadelphia, JB Lippincott, 1975.

Sleisenger MH, Fordtran JS: *Gastrointestinal Disease: Pathophysiology, Diagnosis, Management,* 2nd ed. Philadelphia, WB Saunders, 1978.

Smith DR: *General Urology,* 9th ed. Los Altos, Lange, 1978.

Spark RF, Bikstein G: Bromocriptine and endocrine disorders. *Ann Intern Med* 90:949-956, 1979.

Sparling PF: Diagnosis and treatment of syphilis. *N Engl J Med* 284:642-653, 1971.

Spiro HM: *Clinical Gastroenterology,* 2nd ed. New York, Macmillan, 1977.

Stamey TA: Chronic bacterial prostatitis and the diffusion of drugs into prostatic fluid. *Trans Am Assoc Genitourin Surg* 61:27-34, 1969.

Stanbury JB, Wyngaarden JB, Fredrickson DS: *The Metabolic Basis of Inherited Disease,* 4th ed. New York, McGraw-Hill, 1978.

Stennis BM, Lemola M: Hypersensitivity to ASA and tartrazine in patients with asthma. *Clin Allergy* 6:119-129, 1976.

Sterling L, Reftoff S, Selenknow HA: T_3 thyrotoxicosis. Thyrotoxicosis due to elevated serum triiodothyronine levels. *JAMA* 213:571-575, 1970.

Stiehm ER, Fulginiti VA: *Immunologic Disorders in Infants and Children,* 2nd ed. Philadelphia, WB Saunders, 1980.

Thompson RA: *The Practice of Clinical Immunology,* 2nd ed. Chicago, Year Book Medical, 1978.

Tower DB: *Clinical Neurosciences,* vol 2. New York, Raven Press, 1975.

Tyson JA, Felig P: Medical aspects of diabetes in pregnancy and the diabetogenic effects of oral contraceptives. *Med Clin North Am* 55:947-959, 1971.

Vaughan VC III, McKay RJ, Behrman RE (eds): *Nelson Textbook of Pediatrics,* 11th ed. Philadelphia, WB Saunders, 1979.

Vyas GN, Stites DP, Brecher G: *Laboratory Diagnosis of Immunologic Disorders.* New York, Grune & Stratton, 1975.

Waldvogel FA, Medoff G, Swartz MN: Osteomyelitis: a review and unusual aspects. *N Engl J Med* 282:198-206, 260-266, 316-322, 1970.

Wayne KS: Positive end-expiratory pressure (PEEP) ventilation. *JAMA* 236: 1394-1396, 1976.

Weinstein L, Rubin R: Infective endocarditis. *Prog Cardiovasc Dis* 16:239-264, 1973.

Werner SC, Ingbar SH: *The Thyroid,* 4th ed. Hagerstown, Harper & Row, 1978.

Wilcocks C, Manson-Bahr PE: *Manson's Tropical Diseases,* 17th ed. Baltimore, Williams & Wilkins, 1972.

Winship D, et al: Pancreatitis: pancreatic pseudocysts and their complications. *Gastroenterology* 73:593-603, 1977.

Wortsman J, Soler NG, Hirschowitz J: Cyproheptadine in the management of galactorrhea-amenorrhea syndrome. *Ann Intern Med* 90:923-925, 1980.

Wright R, et al: *Liver and Biliary Disease.* Philadelphia, WB Saunders, 1980.

Youmans GP, Paterson PY: *The Biological and Clinical Basis of Infectious Diseases.* Philadelphia, WB Saunders, 1975.

Yow MD, Baker CJ, Barrett FF, et al: Initial antibiotic management of bacterial meningitis (selection in relationship to age). *Medicine* 52:305-309, 1973.

Yunis JJ, Bloomfield CD, Ensrud K: All patients with acute nonlymphocytic leukemia may have a chromosomal defect. *N Engl J Med* 305:135-139, 1981.